Praise for *Cultured Food for Life*

"*Cultured Food for Life* is just what the doctor should be ordering!
This book is loaded with health wisdom that can change your life!"

— **Christiane Northrup, M.D.,** ob/gyn physician and author of the *New York Times*
bestsellers *Women's Bodies, Women's Wisdom* and *The Wisdom of Menopause*

"Donna Schwenk has taken lacto-fermentation to a whole new level with this attractive
and creative book. She provides plenty of new ideas and some old favorites for the
alchemy of fermented foods. *Cultured Food for Life* is a great contribution to the
growing movement in natural pickling and healthy, digestible grains."

— **Sally Fallon Morell,** author of *Nourishing Traditions* and
president of The Weston A. Price Foundation

"More and more, the research is clear that the true secret to health, vitality, and
weight loss lies in the quality of our intestinal flora. *Cultured Food for Life* is an invaluable
resource for creating that healthy flora in a simple, fun, sustainable, and delicious way. Read
the book, follow the suggestions, enjoy the recipes, and watch how you and your family
experience energy and a vibrancy you've never thought possible."

— **Jon Gabriel,** international best-selling author and creator of The Gabriel Method

"Donna's passion and experience, along with her easy-to-follow recipes,
make this book a must-have for anyone interested in fermented foods."

— **Stepfanie Romine,** co-author of *The SparkPeople Cookbook* and *The Spark Solution*

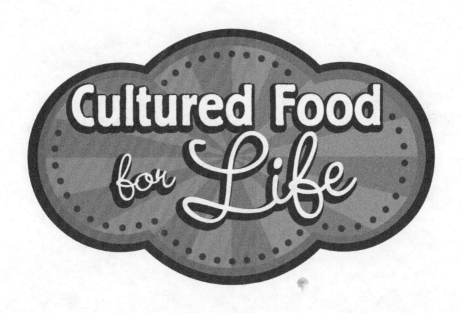

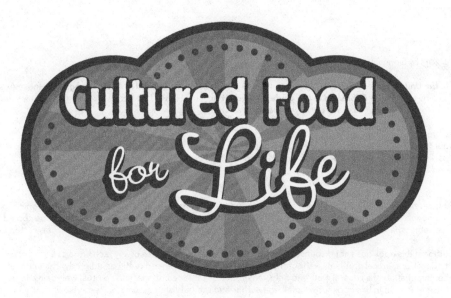

How to Make and Serve Delicious
Probiotic Foods for Better Health and Wellness

DONNA SCHWENK

HAY
HOUSE

Copyright © 2013 by Donna Schwenk

Published in the United States by: Hay House, Inc.: www.hayhouse.com® • **Published in Australia by:** Hay House Australia Pty. Ltd.: www.hayhouse.com.au • **Published in the United Kingdom by:** Hay House UK, Ltd.: www.hayhouse.co.uk • **Published in India by:** Hay House Publishers India: www.hayhouse.co.in

Indexer: Jay Kreider
Cover design: Amy Rose Grigoriou • *Interior design:* Tricia Breidenthal
Insert photos: Donna Schwenk, Maci Schwenk, and Malonda Hutson
Cultured Food Life logo: Shelley Hanna

Library of Congress Cataloging-in-Publication Data

Schwenk, Donna.
  Cultured food for life : how to make and serve delicious probiotic foods for better health and wellness / Donna Schwenk.
    pages cm
  Includes index.
    ISBN 978-1-4019-4282-3 (pbk.) 1. Probiotics. 2. Fermented foods--Recipes. 3. Gastrointestinal system--Microbiology. I. Title.
  RM666.P835S39 2013
  613.2'6--dc23
                                        2013011420

Tradepaper ISBN: 978-1-4019-6945-5

1st edition, October 2013

Printed in the United States of America

*To my daughters, Maci and Holli, who came into
my life to teach me that wisdom was just a prayer away
and that we were truly meant to live a life of joy.
To my son, DJ, the kindest person I know; and to my husband,
Ron, who has been the love of my life for nearly 30 years.
You have all inspired me to be more than I ever thought
I could be. Thanks for filling my life with love!*

CONTENTS

YOUR CULTURED FOOD GUIDE

Dramatically improve your health by eating foods filled with dynamic probiotics that supercharge your body! Join Donna Schwenk at www.culturedfoodlife.com—a special place where you can go to find information and inspiration. Learn not only how to make cultured foods but also how to make them in ways that your entire family will love. There are numerous resources to help you on this new and exciting journey. Check out just a few:

- **Free recipes, articles, and videos**—plus a free *Getting Started Guide* e-book—to help you begin your journey.

- **Hundreds of photos,** including images of most of the foods in this book.

- **Online store** with links to products and ingredients mentioned in this book—and that Donna uses every day when making cultured foods.

- **Donna's DVD, *The Trilogy,*** which contains videos on how to make kefir, kombucha, and cultured vegetables.

- **A community of enthusiasts** who have shared dozens of inspiring testimonials about how cultured foods changed their lives. These are the stories that keep Donna going day after day.

- **Biotic Pro membership** that gives you access to premium content, including exclusive online recipes and hours of quality videos culled from Donna's classes and her home-cooking adventures—there's even one about making cultured foods on a boat. Plus, you can catch "**Donna's Road Map,**" her new series of mini videos that answer all your questions about creating and enjoying cultured foods.

- **Membership Forum** to which, as a Biotic Pro, you'll have access as well as a place where you can ask questions, share your stories, and get help with anything and everything related to cultured foods.

To all of you who've avoided cultured foods, thinking that they're daunting and difficult, visit www.culturedfoodlife.com to find out just how simple it is to incorporate these foods into your life, and to learn how easy they are to prepare.

INTRODUCTION

Welcome to the
World of Cultured Foods

Hi! I'm Donna Schwenk, and I'm here to guide you through a world that seems new and daunting to a lot of people. That's how it was for me not so long ago. It was 2002, and I was sick, tired, miserable, and completely unaware of the power of cultured foods. I needed help, and I found it. And once I learned how life-changing these foods could be, there was no going back. I read book after book. I scoured the Internet. I made it my passion to find out everything I could. Even now, years later, I am continually amazed at the benefits of cultured foods.

As I saw these foods transform my health and my life from the inside out, I knew there was no way I was going to keep this knowledge to myself. Others needed to know, too. *You need to know.* You need to know that it's not normal to always be tired and in pain. If you're like a great many of the people I've met in the classes I teach and through the communities I lead on Facebook and my own website, culturedfoodlife.com, you've forgotten what it feels like to be full of life, looking forward to waking up each morning. That's just where I was, and as I started looking into why, I found some exciting answers—and those answers lie in the gut of the human body with some nonhuman organisms.

good, and we begin to feel the symptoms of disease. But by working to restore a healthy balance to the body's bacteria, and to encourage the good bacteria on a regular basis, we can activate the body's natural tendency for health and well-being. Your body is designed to experience unbelievable wellness and longevity—if you just treat it right. It can give you the chance to live a life of incredible joy. This is all within your power. You no longer have to be one of those people who watches others and wonders what they have that gives them such an advantage.

I know this seems like a big promise, but I truly believe in the power of the body and the bacteria that make it their home. My goal is to bring this knowledge and its benefits to everyone: That's why I started my website. That's why I teach classes. And that's why I was inspired to write this book—and the previous self-published edition. It's also why I work as the Kansas City Chapter leader for the Weston Price Foundation, a worldwide organization comprised of people dedicated to restoring nutrient-dense food to the human diet through education, research, and activism.

This book is part memoir, part how-to guide, and part cookbook. In the pages that follow, I'll cover the cultured foods that have made such a difference in my life and in the lives of my family members, and I'll share some remarkable stories of healing. Let's face it, I've fallen in love with kefir, kombucha, cultured vegetables, and sprouted grains. I eat them every day! And now you can, too. After reading this book, you'll understand the basics of the age-old food preparation technique of fermentation. I'll show you the benefits of cultured foods and how easy and affordable it is to make them at home.

After the introduction to these basics, you can browse through more than 130 recipes to figure out how best to bring these magical foods into your life. I'm sure you'll discover some new dishes, but I'll also show you how to incorporate cultured foods into some of your current favorites. Chocolate waffles, anyone? Finally, this book provides additional resources for buying cultures and equipment as well as for further reading if you want to know more.

By bringing these foods into your life, I have no doubt that you'll begin to feel better soon. I know change can be scary, but if we share the journey, we can get there faster and be successful. So read through this book, and see what makes sense for you. Visit my website and watch my videos. Become a part of the community and the cultured-food movement. I think there is a strong desire to help one another built into our DNA. When

PART I

The Living Food You Should Be Eating

CHAPTER ONE

Coming into Culture

I was 41 years old and holding my new baby in my arms, but it wasn't the beautiful experience I had hoped for. My little one was born seven weeks prematurely and weighed only four pounds—and I was the cause. I had had severe preeclampsia, my liver had started shutting down, and the doctor said that my daughter had to be delivered immediately. This is not how I had imagined the experience. But the signs had been there. The pregnancy wasn't easy, and I had developed gestational diabetes.

But the birth was over, my baby was going to be fine, and my diabetes disappeared. I thought that everything was returning to normal, but several months later, the diabetes returned, and an alarm bell went off in my head. I knew a lot about diabetes—I'd seen it firsthand in my own family and I learned a lot from my friends and family members who work in the medical field. And as I looked at my beautiful baby in my lap, I knew I had to change. I wanted to be vibrant and healthy for this little one, and I knew I couldn't raise her the way I wanted to if I had diabetes. I wanted to live a long life filled with joy and love and family, and if my health didn't change, I realized that this might not happen.

I will never forget that day, sitting in the rocking chair with tears rolling down my cheeks. I cried out from a deep place in my soul for help and wisdom. Little did I know that this baby was coming into my life to save me and to teach me who I really am. Here's what happened: Holli was ten-and-a-half months old when she decided to stop nursing.

six weeks in the womb. Premature babies like Holli don't get that safeguard. When she was born, the hospital staff stressed that the only way to protect her was to nurse her as often as possible for a year or two.

Without the immunity shield, preemies are more susceptible to all kinds of complications from everyday colds and viruses. And as soon as Holli stopped nursing, I witnessed this firsthand. She began having frequent colds and countless sleepless nights. It was hard on both of us. Then one afternoon in a health-food store, I stumbled upon a book called *The Body Ecology Diet* by Donna Gates. I picked up the book and it fell open to a page on kefir and an explanation of kefir's benefits. I was intrigued. The next book on the shelf was *Nourishing Traditions* by Sally Fallon. When I opened that book, I happened to turn to a page on kefir. Just then, a store employee walked by. He stopped, turned to me, and said, "That is the most important book you'll ever read. You should pay attention. It could change everything you thought you knew." Then he just strolled away. I had never heard of kefir, and yet in the space of a few minutes two books had opened to pages on it and a total stranger had told me to pay attention. So I walked over to the dairy section, found the kefir, grabbed a bottle, and put it in my cart—along with those two books. Then I checked out and headed home, quietly hoping that this was the answer to my prayers.

I immediately began to add one to two teaspoons of kefir to each of Holli's bottles. What happened shocked me—in one month my baby had gained four pounds! That's a lot for a preemie. She had color in her cheeks, and she was sleeping through the night. She stopped spitting up everything, and she began to thrive. So we upped her kefir intake, and in a short time, she became the healthiest person in the house.

I started drinking the kefir, too. Not too long after that, I was standing at my kitchen window looking out at the birds and thinking, *They're hungry. I'm going to run out and give them some bird food.* Now you may not think this is a big deal, but when you feel sick and run-down, you don't care about the birds. They can feed themselves. But on this day, something had lifted inside of me, and I felt joy and wellness. This was how I was supposed to feel, and I had forgotten what it was like. My blood pressure was healthy, and my blood sugar numbers had normalized. I became addicted to the good feeling, and I wanted to feel like that every day. This was my beginning. I became a woman on a mission: to discover what had happened to me. What was this kefir and how had it changed Holli and me so dramatically? What was in this ancient food that restored me to my true self?

THE BASIS OF YOUR BODY

Inside each and every one of us there is a whole world of living organisms that, for the most part, go unnoticed and unacknowledged. This is the world of the human gut and its bacteria. Most people are only familiar with bad bacteria—bacteria that cause disease and other negative effects—but did you know that more than 99 percent of bacteria are harmless? And some of these actually prevent disease and keep us healthy? We all have bacteria, and much of your health lies in making sure the good bacteria in your system outnumber the bad. This is a lifelong process that begins at birth.

When you were in your mother's womb, you were in a sterile environment, but when you passed through the birth canal or entered the world through a Cesarean section, you were infused with bacteria from everyone and everywhere—your mother, the doctors, the nurses, the environment—pretty much anyone and anything you came in contact with affected the bacteria in your system. And this is important because it laid the foundation of your inner world. These bacteria are responsible for many of the biological processes that influence your life. They supply us with necessary vitamins and protect us from disease-causing invaders. They break down sugars and proteins and provide us with energy. The breakdown of sugars is basically fermentation that happens in our colon, and the end result is the production of short-chain fatty acids, which do a host of great things.

Short-chain fatty acids prevent overgrowth of pathogenic bacteria like salmonella by making the environment in the large intestine more acidic. They are also phenomenal sources of energy because they're so easily absorbed by the body. If the bacteria in our gut aren't able to break down and process our food into short-chain fatty acids, our bodies simply excrete it without gaining the benefit of the energy the food can provide, which can be up to 10 percent of a healthy individual's daily energy needs.

In addition to the good that comes from short-chain fatty acids, experimental studies also suggest that ingesting healthy bacteria may have other health benefits like lowering blood-sugar and blood-cholesterol levels.[1] Bacteria are also involved in synthesizing hormones and vitamin precursors, plus they're almost entirely responsible for making our body's supply of vitamin B12, a nutrient that supports the health of the body's nerve and blood cells.[2] These are just a few of the millions of things that bacteria do every day inside of you. But they can't do this entirely on their own. It's important to cultivate the good bacteria, so they can crowd out and overpower the toxic ones. That's what cultured foods do. Kefir, kombucha, and cultured vegetables are packed with powerful, beneficial bacteria that enhance the flora in your gut. Ingesting these bacteria leads to colonization and, thus, to a healthy immune force.

Many people wonder if probiotic pills provide the same benefit, as they seem to be marketed in the same way—healthy bacteria for our guts. However, probiotic foods work significantly better because of their construction. To get into the small intestine and colon, where they do the work of breaking down and processing food and powering up the immune system, the bacteria first have to move through the stomach, but the stomach is filled with acid designed to kill bacteria. When you eat a probiotic food, the food itself provides a protective armor that helps shield the friendly bacteria. It also speeds the transport out of the stomach, thus keeping the good bacteria intact. Probiotic pills are often trapped in the acids of the stomach, and the probiotics are killed before the body ever gets a chance to use them. So consuming probiotic foods, such as kefir, kombucha, and cultured vegetables, is much more effective than taking pills.

We are what we eat, and we know, now, that dietary intake greatly influences the types of bacteria in our systems and how they affect us throughout our lives. I saw a huge difference between my two older children who didn't eat probiotic foods as infants and the one who did. My older children struggled with ear infections and doctor's visits due to illness. My youngest daughter, who did receive kefir, has yet to visit a doctor due to illness—and she was the one I was told had a shaky immune system because she was a preemie. I have also seen this in myself. Since I started eating cultured foods, I've been extraordinarily healthy. So I challenge you to open your mind to the good side of bacteria; it far outweighs the bad. It is a whole new world, and one you won't be sorry you've discovered.

So there you have it: a hardy welcome to your inner world! It carries on mostly without your understanding, but longs to work in harmony with you.

EXPERIENCING THE POWER OF CULTURED FOODS

While it's helpful to read about the science behind the benefits people experience when eating cultured foods, the thing that inspires me—and the people I work with—is the

would wake up every morning, drag herself to the kitchen, and say, "Mom. I don't feel good. I never feel good." It broke my heart. She was constantly tired, and suffered the pain and discomfort of general digestive issues. She was unable to eat wheat, and every week the list of foods that hurt her got longer. We took her to doctor after doctor, each of whom came to the conclusion that she was *probably* dealing with irritable bowel syndrome (IBS), but no one was willing to give a strict diagnosis. Finally, one doctor suggested that she needed surgery to remove her gallbladder, but he couldn't give us a reason why. I'm not one of those people who just accepts these things, so we began seeking other help. A kindhearted acupuncturist provided me with an aha moment when he looked at Maci and said, "You have too much hurry and worry, and your body is hurting you because of this." It was true. Our beautiful bodies don't lie—something was out of whack in her life, and we needed to address it. The way I do this is through food.

We had already found kefir, but I hadn't yet discovered the power of all the other cultured foods. When I began researching, I found that these foods were great options for naturally addressing Maci's underlying problem rather than merely treating the symptoms by eliminating certain foods from her diet.

What I discovered was that the lining of Maci's gut was damaged. Stress and a lack of nutrient-dense foods were destroying her: she wasn't getting enough of the right bacteria and enzymes to transform her food into the vitamins and fatty acids that her body needed to stay healthy. Years of antibiotics had stripped her of all her good bacteria, so her food wasn't being processed correctly, and she felt ill because of this. So I started her on a diet that would help bring the desirable bacteria back and heal her gut.

Maci starting eating cultured foods at every meal: kefir for breakfast, one to two tablespoons of cultured veggies at lunch and dinner, and kombucha or coconut kefir to drink at every meal. I also served her a lot of soups made from bone broths. (Bone broths are healing to the digestive tract because of the collagen they contain.) She also took coconut oil by the tablespoon, usually three tablespoons a day. All these foods are healing to the gut, and each one plays a different part in the process. Today, Maci has a fully functioning, pain-free digestive system. She can eat whatever she wants, and she has more energy than you can imagine.

My other favorite story comes from one of my most adamant skeptics. When I first found these foods I was a bit shy about admitting to them. It was hard enough convincing extraordinarily healthy foods. So I didn't really talk about them with other people. Until one day, the dam burst.

Once a week, I have a set date with a group of mothers and their kids. We'd get together, eat lunch, and hang out. This particular day, I was sitting at lunch and looking at the kids in the group: One boy was coughing so much from asthma that he could barely breathe, let alone play. The girl next to him had sores on the sides of her mouth, and she was on a very strict diet because of food allergies. Listening to that boy struggle for breath finally pushed me over the edge. I started talking to his mom about kefir, and how I thought it could help him. Then I talked with the little girl's mom, telling her that I thought cultured foods could heal her daughter's food allergies.

Much to my surprise, they listened—and not only that, they started adding cultured foods into their families' diets. This was my first experience of being privileged to watch people transform their children's lives and their own. And this transformation often steered our lunchtime conversations. Eventually, one of the other mothers decided that she was tired of listening to all this talk about cultured foods, and she stopped sitting with the group, accusing us of having a food cult. It was pretty funny, but I can imagine that it does sound a little weird if you haven't experienced cultured foods.

At the point when she abandoned our table, she was pregnant. Sadly, after her son was born, he didn't thrive: he was terribly thin and could barely tolerate breast milk, and he wasn't functioning up to his age level in other measurements of development. As he grew, he continued to struggle. He was in physical therapy, occupational therapy, and play therapy. He was allergic to everything, and went through test after test with an allergist and worked with a dietician. He couldn't form sentences, so he also had a speech therapist. And he had vision problems. Life was rough, and it was heartbreaking to see.

Finally, as a last resort, his mom came to me. She remembered the talk of cultured foods and the improvements they made in the lives of those at our table of "food cultists." She began sprouting grains and making kefir, kombucha, and lots of cultured veggies. She started with coconut kefir because her son was allergic to dairy, and what happened was nothing short of astounding. I'll let her tell you what happened:

> Donna, this is so emotional! I can't believe I am the mother of a miracle—and yes, I truly believe he is! After all we've been through, I never expected my son to walk or talk or

time. But he was taking it in! He was storing all that info for later! I wanted to let you know that the little brain that wasn't able to talk for the longest time and just gazed around like he couldn't comprehend anything—*that* little brain *is reading!!! At three years old!* I kid you not, Donna! I think he will start piano lessons soon—he *loves* music.

The other day, I decided that since we ran out of coconut milk, we might as well go with raw milk. And he did great. *I am thrilled!!!* I can't tell you how big of a breakthrough this is for us! I even gave him raw milk and his sprouted cookies for a snack today! It has been a very hard road for us, and we are still on it, but our road has been made so much smoother because of your help! *Thank you, thank you, thank you* for your help and for never tiring of my scoffing!

I am continually inspired by stories I hear and the well-being I see in the people I know and love. These foods do the work, and you receive the benefits. I never had any intention of writing a book or teaching classes or having a website and a blog. But as Joseph Campbell said, "We must be willing to let go of the life we have planned, so as to accept the one that is waiting for us."

SHARING THE WEALTH

Beginning a life with cultured foods is a personal journey. I began with kefir, but you may choose to start somewhere else. Whatever you choose is great, but there are some practicalities that you should know about before you begin.

From what I've seen and experienced, the best way to start adding cultured foods into your life is to do so slowly. These are very powerful detoxification agents, and many people experience some unpleasant symptoms if they move full speed ahead. They experience what is known as a Herxheimer Reaction. Herxing is believed to occur when injured or dead bacteria release their toxins into the blood and tissues faster than the body can comfortably handle. The immune system's response is sudden, exaggerated inflammation, which you may endure as gastrointestinal distress, stomachaches, headaches, skin rashes, diarrhea, constipation, or other flulike symptoms. These symptoms are generally short-lived, and they won't necessarily happen to you. As it turns out, the more toxic your gut, the more symptomatic you'll be. But this is good, because it means that your body is de-

When I advise people at the beginning of their journey, I suggest that they choose whichever cultured food—kefir, kombucha, or cultured veggies—is most appealing, and start there. Eat or drink just a bit of the cultured food each day, and pay attention to the effects that it has on your body. If you don't notice anything, feel free to consume more of the same food. If you are having symptoms, just keep taking small portions until your body stabilizes. Generally, I recommend that you stick to just one food type for at least a week before you add in another category. The goal is to get all three cultured foods—plus sprouted grains—into your daily diet. When people consume all these foods every day, they see the biggest differences. It's the combination of the different bacteria in each cultured food that makes the body thrive. This is what happened in my life and my family's. We would get better as we consumed one cultured food, but our health skyrocketed when we added all three to our daily lives. And through the years, I've seen the same thing happen to hundreds of other people.

So how much do you begin with? Here are my recommendations:

- **Kefir:** Consume one-quarter to one-half cup of kefir daily. If you experience gassy or flulike symptoms, back off and have kefir every other day until the body adjusts. If you don't have any symptoms, increase the amount you are drinking to one cup of kefir daily. You can make this into a smoothie or a pudding, or use a recipe in Part II or on my site for variety.

- **Cultured Veggies:** Add one tablespoon of cultured veggies to both lunch and dinner. Once again, if you have side effects that are uncomfortable, back off and eat the vegetables every other day until your body adjusts.

- **Kombucha:** Start out by drinking four ounces a day. If you have any symptoms, drink it every other day until they subside.

Once your body adjusts to cultured foods, I say, the more, the better! I no longer think of them as some sort of "medicine" to be taken at a prescribed dosage or at a particular time of day. Now I simply love them, and I fit as many healthy bacteria into my daily diet and my family's as I can. Over time, I've found many different ways to incorporate cultured foods into our favorite dishes; I've also experimented with flavors, creating delicious drinks like kefir smoothies and kombucha "cocktails." Even my daughter Maci has become a cultured food connoisseur, she loves cooking with them, and you'll find many of her reci

CHAPTER TWO

Meet My Friend Kefir

I am pleased to introduce you to my good friend kefir, pronounced either KEE-fur or kuh-FEER, depending on whom you ask. Kefir is a fermented milk drink that has been around for thousands of years. Because of its long history, there are many claims and legends associated with it: People in the Caucasus Mountains maintain that kefir is the reason for their legendary longevity. In Turkey, scrolls from Abraham declared that his long life was due to fermented milk products. Muhammad professed that kefir grains were a gift from Allah to him. And Noah claimed to have gotten these grains from angels on the ark. Whatever the case, you can see the common theme: kefir makes you healthy and aids in longevity. It's no surprise that the word *kefir* is said to have originated from the Turkish word *keif*, which means "good feeling."

The consistency of kefir is creamy, sometimes bubbly, and similar to pourable yogurt. But kefir is *not* yogurt. Homemade kefir has between 30 and 56 strains of good bacteria, while yogurt has only 7 to 10. And the types of bacteria in kefir are also quite different from those in yogurt. The bacteria in yogurt pass through the body within 24 hours, their main purpose being to sustain the good bacteria that already reside in the digestive system. Kefir, however, is a source of those good bacteria. The bacteria in kefir stay and take up residence, creating a colony that remains in the digestive system.

Health Benefits of Kefir

What seems like ages ago when I was battling high blood pressure and diabetes, I noticed an interesting trend in my body. It seemed that when I drank a glass of kefir every day, my blood pressure would go down—and not just a little bit. It would drop significantly, putting me back within the normal range. When I would skip my kefir, my blood pressure would start creeping back up within three days or so.

I know that jumping to conclusions is wrong, because there are so many other variables, so I started doing experiments on myself to see if it was truly the kefir that was making the difference. After many trial runs, I was convinced that it was the kefir that was healing me. A couple of months later, my personal experience was backed up in a book I was reading, *Bacteria for Breakfast* by Dr. Kelly Downhower Karpa. This book discusses fermented milk products and their ability to lower blood pressure in people with mild hypertension. It includes the results of a study involving both rats and human subjects that confirmed Dr. Karpa's findings.[3] To combat hypertension, doctors often prescribe what is known as an ACE-inhibitor, a drug that dilates the blood vessels, resulting in lower blood pressure. The study reviewed in *Bacteria for Breakfast* found that some strains of probiotic food produce their own ACE-inhibiting substances during the fermentation process.

While most bacteria produce lactic acid, they also produce ACE-inhibiting substances during milk fermentation; *Lactobacillus helveticus,* which is found in high concentrations in kefir, was identified as the most effective. However, it is important to note that the results were most effective for patients with mild hypertension. I am not advising anyone to stop taking medication, but it may be beneficial to add some kefir to your diet, and then monitor yourself to see if you experience a lowering of your blood pressure.

Kefir also has properties that assist in controlling blood sugar, because it's loaded with lactic acid and enzymes that regulate sugar metabolism.[4] My blood sugars quickly fell into the normal range when I added kefir to my diet. It was quite miraculous to me—and I have noticed this phenomenon in others who attended my cultured-food classes.

3 V. Usta et al. "A Placebo-Controlled Study of the Effect of Sour Milk on Blood Pressure in Hypertensive Subjects"

Another benefit of kefir is that the types of bacteria it contains help alleviate inflammation throughout the gut.[5] Controlling inflammation is critical, because many diseases are caused or affected by it. If your body's ability to regulate inflammation is not working properly, you're headed toward illness and premature aging.

Finally, kefir enhances digestion because its milk sugars have been predigested through the fermentation process, making it extremely low in sugar: kefir is only 1 percent sugar, while yogurt is 4 percent.

This predigestion also helps regulate the immune system's response, leading to less stress throughout the body. In a study that used a diabetes-prone breed of mice, researchers investigated whether or not the administration of *Lactobacillus casei*—one of the probiotic bacteria found in abundance in kefir—would prevent these mice from developing diabetes when the disease was induced. The progression into diabetes in the mice mimics the onset of human insulin-dependent diabetes mellitus. Researchers found that the administration of this strain of bacteria did, indeed, reduce the development of diabetes in these mice by regulating immune responses. The exact mechanisms by which these actions prevent diabetes are yet to be understood.[6]

Although there are few rigorous studies on the health benefits of kefir, there are many advantages reported by those people who drink it on a regular basis. In my classes and on my websites, I've received many stories of miraclelike healing, but they still bowl me over. In addition to those benefits listed above, here are some of the most common reports about what kefir has done for people—and some of these, I've even experienced myself:

- Eliminates constipation

- Reduces or eliminates allergies

- Enhances digestion

- Reduces or eliminates asthma symptoms

- Reduces or eliminates cold and flu illnesses

- Cures acne

- Treats yeast infections

5 A.L. Hart, A.J. Stagg, and M.A. Kamm. "Use of Probiotics in the Treatment of Inflammatory Bowel Disease," *Journal*

- Promotes a natural "good" feeling
- Effective as the strongest natural antibiotic without side effects
- Replenishes the body with good bacteria after antibiotic use
- Treats diarrhea
- Aids lactose intolerance
- Promotes deep sleep
- Heals ulcers

The kefir-drinking community that I interact with on a daily basis talks about these benefits—not the scientific community. But there are so many stories of people who have been helped by kefir that I have no doubt about its health-enhancing effects. One of my favorites came from a woman who learned about kefir in one of my classes. Several weeks later, she e-mailed me an extraordinary story of how kefir came to the aid of her husband. He had been diagnosed with a rare disease that gave him intense stomach pain when he ate solid foods. His only recourse was to puree everything. After drinking kefir for a few weeks, he was able to eat normally again with no pain! I hope you are able to experience wonderful things in your life, too!

Bringing Kefir into Your Life

I started my life with kefir by drinking Lifeway kefir, a brand that comes in a variety of wonderful flavors and that can be found in health-food stores and many large grocery stores. When kefir and I got more serious, I bought kefir culture starter packets, so I could start making my own. And finally, I purchased living kefir grains, and have been preparing kefir with these ever since.

I experienced great breakthroughs from all these sources of kefir, and I still buy Lifeway if I'm really busy or in need of one of their unique flavors. But I now ferment my own kefir, because the store-bought variety has only a fraction of the bacterial strains—10 for the retail type as compared to 30 to 56 for homemade. It's also much less expensive to make it, plus you can customize the flavors to suit your personal taste. I'm not the kind of

Making Kefir

There are two ways to make kefir. You can use live kefir grains that reproduce and will last a lifetime if you treat them right (I've had mine for more than 11 years!), or you can purchase kefir freeze-dried culture packets. A starter package of six freeze-dried culture packets will produce 42 gallons of kefir, and the instructions are included. In the recipe for Basic Kefir, I teach you how to make kefir using live grains.

If you're not lucky enough to have a friend with grains to spare, kefir grains can be purchased from a number of reliable sources (see Resources, page 208). These kefir grains will eagerly transform your milk into something even healthier for you. I personally recommend raw (unpasteurized) goat's or cow's milk for the maximum benefits, but as raw milk isn't available everywhere, it's fine to use pasteurized whole milk. Skim and low-fat milk—as well as almond or coconut milk—also work, but whole milk provides the most food for the grains. Do not use ultra-pasteurized or lactose-free milk. And never heat your grains or place them in a jar still hot from the dishwasher. Heat and lack of food are the two things that will kill kefir grains.

One concern I often hear from people just beginning to make their own kefir is their worry about having left their kefir out for too long. This is not something to fret over. However, don't leave the kefir out for more than a couple of days, because the grains will need nourishment, and if they go too long without it, they'll die. The longer the kefir is at room tem-

BASIC KEFIR

You can use the method below to make any amount of kefir you desire; just keep in mind that a good rule of thumb is to use 1 tablespoon of kefir grains per 1 cup of milk. So, if you want to make 1 cup of kefir, use 1 tablespoon of kefir grains and 1 cup of milk. For 2 cups of kefir, use 2 tablespoons of kefir grains and 2 cups of milk. And so on.

Step 1: Place the kefir grains in a glass jar that can be securely sealed. I like canning jars with plastic lids, but you can use any jar that will close securely.

Step 2: Using the 1 tablespoon to 1 cup ratio of kefir grains to milk, add the appropriate amount of milk to the jar.

Step 3: Securely seal the jar, and leave it on your kitchen counter, out of direct sunlight, or in a cabinet at room temperature for 24 hours.

Step 4: After 24 hours, remove the kefir grains using a slotted spoon or a mesh strainer. (The strainer can be stainless steel or plastic.) Add the kefir grains to fresh milk to begin another fermentation or for storage (see page 17).

Step 5: Transfer the strained kefir to your

grains in the milk to ferment for several days. But to me, that makes it too sour. Kefir should be enjoyed, and the better it tastes, the more you'll drink.

Second-Fermented Kefir

Many years ago, I discovered that a second fermentation not only makes kefir taste better, but also increases its nutrients. It is now the only way I make my kefir! Second fermenting isn't difficult, and it reduces some of the sour taste of the kefir. The process also increases certain B vitamins, like folic acid, and makes the calcium and magnesium more bioavailable (meaning that your body can take in more of the nutrients and use them immediately).

Second fermenting your kefir can be done with almost any fruit or spice. Basically, it entails adding a flavor of your choosing to kefir, sealing the container, and letting it sit at room temperature for another 24 hours. I have second fermented my kefir using all sorts of different flavorings, from cinnamon sticks and orange peel to chai tea and strawberries and blueberries. To get the intensity of flavor you want, it often takes some experimentation. For example, when I first used a chai tea bag, I let it ferment for a full 24 hours; however, the chai flavor ended up being too strong, so on the next batch, I left it at room temperature for only 12 hours, and it was perfect! For second fermenting with fruit, I generally recommend that you use about one-quarter to one-half cup of your chosen fruit for the first attempt. You can add more or less for the next batch depending on how you like it. You can even use just

SECOND-FERMENTED CITRUS KEFIR

2 cups Basic Kefir (page 15)

1 organic orange or lemon (see Note)

....

Step 1: Place the kefir in a glass jar that can be securely sealed.

Step 2: Using a vegetable peeler, peel one strip of zest from the orange or lemon—the equivalent of one time around the fruit—avoiding the white pith, which is bitter.

Step 3: Place the zest in the jar with the kefir and close securely.

Step 4: Leave the jar on your kitchen counter, out of direct sunlight, for 24 hours to ferment a second time.

Step 5: After 24 hours, transfer the jar to the

you can check out my post about second-ferment kefirs at www.culturedfoodlife.com/how-to-second-ferment-kefir.

The recipe for Second-Fermented Citrus Kefir (on the previous page) is one of my favorites.

Kefir Cheese and Kefir Whey

Once you love kefir like I do, you'll be on the lookout for more ways to enjoy it. The basic recipe for kefir cheese and whey (in the box below) is where I start with many of the recipes in this book. It's easy to make, and you can flavor the cheese with herbs and spices to make a nice dip or spread like Garlic–Kefir Cheese Dip on page 69. You can also use it plain as you would use cream cheese. The whey that you collect can be used for making fermented drinks or cultured vegetables. Nothing is wasted!

Caring for Your Kefir Grains

As I've already mentioned, kefir grains are alive, and to keep them that way, you have to keep them away from heat and supply them with plenty of food. If you want to take a break from making kefir for more than one or two days, you need to care for your grains in a specific way.

Step 1: Place your kefir grains in fresh milk. Keep in mind the ratio rule of 1 tablespoon of grains to 1 cup of milk.

Step 2: Place this jar of kefir grains and milk in the refrigerator.

With this ratio of milk to grains, the grains will stay alive for one week in the refrigerator. If you are going to be gone for more than one week, simply multiply the amount of milk by the numbers of

---

KEFIR CHEESE AND KEFIR WHEY

Makes 1 cup kefir cheese and 1 cup kefir whey

2 cups Basic Kefir (page 15)

Step 1: Place a basket-style coffee filter in a strainer and set the strainer over a bowl.

Step 2: Pour the kefir into the coffee filter. Cover the bowl with plastic wrap and place it in the refrigerator overnight. The bowl will catch the liquid whey, which you can store for future

When you return to making kefir, the milk you drain from the stored kefir grains is not really kefir. It's been kept at too low a temperature in the fridge to ferment properly. I just discard this milk.

OTHER KINDS OF KEFIR

Generally, when people talk about kefir, they are referring to the dairy kefir that we've been discussing until now, but there are other kinds of kefir that I often get asked about—especially by people who are allergic to dairy. The first is almond- or coconut-milk kefir; the other is water kefir.

BASIC ALMOND- OR COCONUT-MILK KEFIR

You can use the method below to make any amount of kefir you desire, just keep in mind that a good rule of thumb is to use the same ratio of grains to milk as for dairy kefir: 1 tablespoon of kefir grains per 1 cup of milk. So if you want to make 1 cup of kefir, use 1 tablespoon of kefir grains and 1 cup of milk. For 2 cups of kefir, use 2 tablespoons of kefir grains and 2 cups of milk. And so on.

Step 1: Place the kefir grains in a glass jar that can be securely sealed. I like canning jars with plastic lids, but you can use any jar that will close securely.

Step 2: Using the 1 tablespoon to 1 cup ratio of kefir grains to milk, add the appropriate amount of almond or coconut milk to the jar.

Step 3: Securely seal the jar, and leave the jar on your kitchen counter, out of direct sunlight, or in a cabinet at room temperature for 18 to 24 hours. Almond or coconut milk will culture

Almond- or Coconut-Milk Kefir

Almond- or coconut-milk kefir is a great alternative to dairy kefir if you are avoiding dairy for any reason. These kefirs have similar benefits to dairy kefir—though the amounts of calcium or magnesium can differ depending on the milk you use. Their probiotic content is just as high, and they also contain super-charged vitamin quantities. However, there are special considerations that you have to take when making almond or coconut kefir. Kefir grains do not survive in almond or coconut milk long term. They grow and thrive by eating the lactose from dairy milk, and since there is no lactose in almond or coconut milk, the grains will need to be refreshed in dairy milk once a week or more. Leave

almond or coconut kefir again. The more often you do this, the more your grains will grow and multiply. It's the lactose that keeps the bacteria alive and thriving.

Remember to refresh the grains each week by making dairy kefir at least once a week. And if you are going to store them or take a break from making kefir, it is best to store the grains in whole dairy milk. Follow the instructions for storing kefir grains on page 17.

Water Kefir

Water kefir is another type of nondairy kefir that is gaining in popularity. Many people start with this method of making kefir because it's so easy and fun. It's made with fruit or vegetable juice or coconut water or an extract, or even just sugar and water. Then a culture is added and the mixture is fermented. Just like in dairy kefir, the good bacteria eat the sugars out of the juice and create probiotics, plus they unlock additional vitamins and minerals. I can't say enough about these water kefirs—or what I refer to as *kefir sodas*—as a replacement for store-bought sodas. In addition to the probiotics, the kefir in the soda eats much of the sugar, so you don't have to deal with the adverse effects of sugar that soda often promotes, like blood-sugar fluctuations and cravings for sweets. There are no chemicals or artificial ingredients in kefir soda. And as a bonus to those of us who crave bubblicious beverages, the kefir creates naturally occurring carbonation.

While I stand by these as a great replacement for store-bought soda, I also want to let you know that of all the cultured foods, this is the one I least recommend. I've learned a few things from my own experience. You can then decide for yourself what's right for you.

First and foremost, there are only 10 strains of good bacteria in water kefir versus 36 to 50 in basic homemade milk kefir. Also, it does not have the high amounts of calcium and magnesium found in dairy kefir.

For people who have problems with *Candida* or diabetes, there is often too much remaining sugar if the soda has not fermented properly. Because it is made with fruit juice or sugar water, you must be sure to let it ferment fully to reduce the sugar content.

The other occasional problem occurs when people have used straight juice to make water kefir. Juice turns to alcohol when you ferment it, so it's important to always dilute the juice with water. I create a half-juice-half-water mixture, and then I ferment it for a minimal

So have I sufficiently scared you? I didn't mean to. I really love water kefir, but I always want to be totally honest with you when relating my experiences. I don't recommend things I haven't tried. I feel that my years of experience are a wonderful asset in helping you bring these wonderful foods into your life, and that means telling you about the good and the bad. I want you to know you can trust me because I will always tell you the truth. It's just how I roll. We're all in this together, helping one another, and that makes it easier on the journey.

Making Kefir Sodas

Kefir sodas can be created in three different ways using three different cultures: kefir whey, water kefir crystals, or kefir culture starter powder (see Resources, page 208). My preference for making kefir sodas is to use the kefir powder because I can reserve a portion of the final product to start a new batch of soda that will ferment faster, thus being available more quickly for my enjoyment.

Kefir Whey Method: Use ½ cup of fresh Kefir Whey (page 17) for each 1-pint (16-ounce) bottle. After mixing the culture with the soda ingredients, seal the bottle and set it on your counter, out of direct sunlight, for approximately 5 days. Check it occasionally to judge the carbonation level. Once it is bubbly enough for you, transfer the bottle to the fridge. Make sure your kefir whey is fresh or it won't culture properly.

Water Kefir Crystal Method: You will need to get a starter box of water kefir crystals to make kefir soda using this method. You can find these crystals on my site, www.culturedfoodlife.com, by clicking the Get Starter Cultures button. One box will last a lifetime. When working with water crystals, do not use bottles. Use a canning jar with a lid, so you can easily remove the crystals at the end of the process. To make the soda, you will need 1 rehydrated box of crystals per 1-pint (16-ounce) container of soda. After mixing the culture with the soda ingredients, seal the jar and set it on your kitchen counter, out of direct sunlight, for 1 to 2 days. Check it occasionally to judge the carbonation level. Once it is bubbly enough for you, remove the water kefir crystals and place the soda in the fridge. Water kefir crystals need to be fed again with some sugar water or fruit juice to be kept alive. For more information on storing water kefir crystals, see page 22.

Powder Method: This is the method I use in most of the kefir soda recipes in Part II. To make kefir soda using the kefir culture starter powder, use ½ packet of powder per 1-pint (16-ounce) bottle. After mixing the culture with the soda ingredients, seal the bottle, and set it on your kitchen counter, out of direct sunlight, for approximately 2 to 3 days. Check it occasionally to judge the carbonation level. Once it is bubbly enough for you, transfer the bottle to the fridge.

When using this method, make sure to reserve some of your finished mixture to start a new batch of soda. You will save about ¼ cup per 1-pint (16-ounce) bottle. Simply put this finished soda into another 1-pint bottle and add fresh juice ingredients. Seal the bottle securely, and let it sit on your counter, out of direct sunlight, for about a day. This second batch—and each subsequent batch—will ferment more quickly than the first batch. You can continue this process until the new soda no longer gets bubbly. At that point, you will need fresh culture starter. One kefir culture starter powder packet has made me as many as 25 quarts of soda.

In the recipes in Part II of this book, I've given instructions using the powder method (unless otherwise noted), along with information about making subsequent batches using reserved soda from the first. When using kefir whey or water kefir crystals, the process starts "fresh" for each batch.

If you prefer to use the kefir whey method or the water kefir crystal method, simply switch out the culture ingredients and make the soda according to the above instructions.

So there you have it! You now know everything you need to know about starting your own life with kefir.

FREQUENTLY ASKED QUESTIONS ABOUT KEFIR

Why is my milk kefir starting to separate and curdle?

It has cultured faster than expected. This is not a bad thing. It just means that your kefir is ready. Remove the grains, and shake or stir the kefir to mix it together again.

Why is my milk kefir culturing so fast and how do I fix it?

This happens for one of two reasons: Your grains have grown, but the amount of milk you're using hasn't increased; or your kitchen is quite warm. If the former, either remove some of the grains or add more milk for the next batch, so the grains to milk ratio remains correct. If a too-cozy kitchen is the problem, reduce

I left my milk kefir grains in the refrigerator for a few months. Are they still good?

Probably not. Kefir grains eat the milk sugars (lactose) out of the milk to live and to make their bacteria. This is why the milk gets more sour. When the grains run out of food, they begin to die. They're living organisms and need food. Treat them like a pet and make sure you feed them.

I stored my milk kefir grains in the fridge for a week. Is the milk that the grains were stored in okay to drink?

The milk that the grains were stored in is not really kefir. It won't hurt you to drink it, but it probably won't taste very good. Milk needs to culture at a warmer temperature to really turn into kefir.

Do I culture milk kefir with a lid or with cheesecloth?

I always culture my kefir with a lid on. I use a one-quart glass canning jar with a plastic lid, but a metal lid is also fine.

Why aren't my milk kefir grains growing?

If you are making kefir every day, your grains should be growing and multiplying. If they aren't, it is because the temperature in your house is cooler than usual, slowing down the grains, or your kefir grains have died. If your milk is turning into kefir by becoming sour and thick, your grains are still working, just at a slower rate. You can purchase more or get some new grains from a friend.

How do I know if my milk kefir grains are still good?

They will culture your milk and turn it sour and thick within 24 to 48 hours. Make sure that you have enough grains for the amount of milk that you are using.

Can I take a break from water kefir?

To take a break from making water kefir, prepare a sugar-water solution, place the crystals in the sugar water, place a tight lid on the container, and place it in the refrigerator. This will keep for a couple of weeks in your fridge. After that, you need to replace the solution with fresh water and sugar. For each one-quarter cup of water kefir crystals, you will need to use one-quarter cup of sugar and one quart of water for the sugar-water solution.

What do I do if my water kefir crystals are slimy and smell bad?

This is usually a result of overcrowding and lack of minerals. Water kefir needs sugar and minerals to culture properly. Add a few drops of liquid mineral supplement, such as the one on my site in the Store, along with sugar to refresh your crystals.

What amount of kefir crystals do I need to make water kefir?

You'll need three to four tablespoons of kefir crystals to culture one to three quarts of water kefir every

CHAPTER THREE

Kombucha: A Magical Tea

After I mastered the art of making and eating kefir, I moved on to another cultured food that I had heard about: kombucha. This fermented tea has been embraced by entire communities who drink it for its preventative and curative effects, so of course, I had to check it out. And since I started drinking it, I've become an intensely loyal and devoted kombucha advocate. I'm shocked at how much love I can feel for a beverage!

Kombucha—pronounced Kom-BOO-cha—is a living health drink that's made by fermenting tea and sugar with a kombucha culture (a combination of bacteria and yeast). The kombucha culture is not pretty. In fact, I've heard it described as looking like a brain, a placenta, or a "sludgy" mass. Not that *sludgy* is a word, but it fits. The culture actually looks somewhat like a large, shiny pancake. While it's not pretty, I think it's beautiful.

You'll hear a lot of names for the kombucha culture, including *mother of vinegar* and *mushroom*, though it is not a fungi at all. The term *kombucha mushroom* probably comes from a misinterpretation of the original Chinese name, which translates to "Tibetan mushroom." In this book, I refer to it as SCOBY, one of the other more common terms you'll run into. This is simply an acronym for *symbiotic culture of bacteria and yeast*.

If you are concerned that kombucha is made with sugar, you needn't be. The sugar is consumed by the culture, leaving a deliciously tart drink. It's not what you would imagine fermented tea would taste like: the result can be something between sparkling apple cider

HEALTH BENEFITS OF KOMBUCHA

Kombucha has been a "secret formula" for those in the know, and it's been considered a lifesaver by many a poor person in the less blessed nations for hundreds of years. Kombucha is full of glucuronic acid, which plays a part in one of the body's most important detoxification processes in which glucuronic acid binds to toxins and transforms them so they can be easily eliminated by the kidneys. The liver produces this substance naturally, but sometimes the body can't keep up with the number of pollutants that it comes into contact with. The extra glucuronic acid in kombucha helps make up the difference.[7]

I would never have believed that kombucha was such a powerful detoxifier if it were not for my own experience. When I started to drink it, the kombucha kicked in immediately. First, I noticed how often I was going to the bathroom, and then I began to smell. The skin is the body's largest elimination organ, and it was doing its job on me. (My daughter had a similar experience.) Luckily, it only lasted a week—and at the end of it, I had the unexpected benefit of not needing to use deodorant. Bad bacteria are the cause of body odor, and I now ingest so much good bacteria that I just don't need it anymore!

The other benefits of kombucha include its oodles of B vitamins and amino acids. B vitamins are some of those very important raw materials that make your body work. B vitamins, which are often called the "happy" vitamins, bring balance to the systems running your body. They convert food to energy and help form healthy red blood cells to reduce or eliminate anemia, among many other functions. Amino acids are the building blocks of the proteins found in our bodies. The human body can produce 10 of its necessary 20 amino acids, but the other 10, which are called essential amino acids, can only be obtained by eating the right foods. When the body doesn't get enough of these essential compounds, it will begin to break down its proteins in search of the nutrients it needs. Kombucha contains many of these essential amino acids.

These are just some of the items that science has begun to study. However, in my personal life, I use kombucha to address many issues. Between my life experiences and those of the people in my classes and community, I've heard of all sorts of benefits.

- Detoxifying the liver to feel healthier and livelier
- Helping quell wracking coughs during cold and flu season

- Relieving headaches and migraines

- Improving digestion

- Relieving seasonal allergies

- Suppressing the appetite for weight loss

- Speeding the healing of ulcers (kombucha kills *h. pylori*, a common ulcer-causing bacterium)

- Boosting energy

- Fortifying the immune system

- Easing joint pain

- Getting rid of yeast problems

The most interesting health benefit I've seen in my own life associated with kombucha has to do with my husband, Ron. Ron has become accustomed to the enthusiasm I express for my discoveries, and he always goes along for the ride, but never jumps in with both feet until coaxed.

Ron had a terrible problem with the glare from headlights and other lighting and had a hard time driving at night. He finally went to an eye doctor and was diagnosed with cataracts. I didn't know until then that there are different kinds of cataracts, and he had the type that develops quickly over a three- to six-month period. The doctor advised that the only way to deal with the cataracts was surgery. He also noted that a cataract was beginning in the other eye, and Ron would probably need a second surgery in the next three to six months. My husband was not happy. He was only 40, but he felt like 90. It was awful to be so young and yet need this surgery so closely associated with the elderly. Medical professionals don't know why it happens—"It just does."

While we didn't know why the cataracts occurred, I knew deep inside that there must be something we could do. In my research, I read that kombucha was great for cataract prevention, so I decided to start there.[8] I made some kombucha, told Ron about my research, and handed him a glass. Much to my surprise, he loved it and started drinking it every day. I was very excited. He would also drink kefir as long as I made it into a smoothie.

Ron had the surgery for the existing cataracts, but he was not a happy camper. Then

"Huh, it stopped. What would make that cataract stop growing? I've never seen anything like that. Huh!" Fast-forward seven years, and it is still the same. He's never had surgery in the other eye, and he's a faithful daily drinker of kombucha.

Clearly, this isn't proof that kombucha stops cataracts, but this addition to his diet was the biggest change he made at that point in his life. This leads me to believe that it played a major part in his eye health. The body is constantly striving to heal itself; kombucha helps bring your body back into balance, so that it may do so naturally.

Bringing Kombucha into Your Life

One of the easiest ways to get kombucha is to buy it at your local health-food store. Look for it in the refrigerated section. There are several brands, but my favorite is GT's Synergy Kombucha—they have so many delicious flavors! While I do make my own kombucha at home, I often grab one from the store when I'm on the go and need a quick pick-me-up.

I decided to start home brewing kombucha, because when you drink as much as my family does, it's a lot less expensive to make it, and homemade is always the best. And it's not difficult to do—almost like making vinegar—and much easier than home brewing beer! By making your own kombucha, you can develop a personalized brew that suits your taste. I've come up with so many interesting versions of this drink that there's something to please every palate. I've also figured out some great ways to incorporate kombucha into salad dressings and other beverages, so the health benefits go even farther. You'll find some of my favorite concoctions in the recipe section.

The amazing feeling I get from kombucha and its bubbly effervescence made me realize the spiritual nature of what we eat and drink. These foods and beverages change you from the inside out. They talk to your genes and become a part of you. Kombucha made me feel so good that I couldn't help but feel more kindness and love toward others. Yes, I am proud to tell you about my friend kombucha. I hope you love it, too. It makes my heart sing every day.

Making Kombucha

- One-gallon glass jug or nonlead-based crock
- Breathable cloth napkin that will fit completely over the top of the jug or crock
- Rubber band to go around the neck of your jug or crock
- Starter

When I say a *starter*, I mean that you will need a kombucha SCOBY and one cup of brewed kombucha tea. If you have a friend who makes kombucha, I'm certain they have a SCOBY to spare, since a new one forms each time kombucha is brewed. I have so many that I don't know what to do with them—I've been feeding them to my friend's chickens, using them as fertilizer in my garden, giving them to friends, and so on. Everyone—plant and animal—loves them! If you don't have a friend who makes kombucha, you can get a starter kit through my website, www.culturedfoodlife.com, or you can check out other options in the Resources section (page 208) of this book. Whatever kit you get should come with one SCOBY and one cup of fermented tea.

The next point I want to make concerns sugar. You'll see in the recipe below that I list three types of sugar: Sucanat, white sugar, and coconut sugar. Sucanat is a brand of pure dried sugar-cane juice. Because it is minimally processed, it retains the nutrients that are removed from white sugar in the refining process. It also contains less sucrose than refined sugar. However, it does have a slight maple or barley taste, so it's not for everyone. I use coconut sugar when I make kombucha, because I like the flavor and the minerals it provides. But if you can't find either of these options, or if they don't appeal to you, you can use plain white sugar—it gets eaten and processed by the bacteria in the culture, so you needn't worry.

The last thing to discuss is the type of tea to use. I've noted in the recipe to use black or green tea, but honestly, any type of tea (or combination of teas) will work. I've used white, jasmine, and rooibos teas, and they all make a delicious kombucha—you just have to figure out which one you prefer. I do not recommend herbal teas or fruit-flavored teas with oils, as they contain antibacterial qualities that could affect the outcome of your kombucha.

BASIC KOMBUCHA

A note before you begin: At the end of this process, you will have created your very own SCOBY. Make sure to keep this—plus one cup of the kombucha you've made—to use as the starter for your next batch.

Makes 3 quarts

3 quarts filtered water (not distilled)

1 cup Sucanat, white sugar, or coconut sugar

4 to 5 tea bags (organic green tea is preferred, but black tea is good, too)

1 SCOBY

1 cup fermented kombucha tea

....

Step 1: Wash all the utensils with hot soapy water and rinse well.

Step 2: Bring the filtered water to a boil in a large pot over medium high heat. When the water has reached a rolling boil, add the sugar and continue to boil for 5 minutes.

Step 3: Turn off the heat and add the tea bags. Steep for 10 to 15 minutes, then remove the tea bags, and let the tea cool to room temperature.

Step 4: Pour the cool tea into the 1-gallon container.

Step 5: Add the SCOBY, placing it so that the smooth shiny surface faces up.

Step 6: Add the fermented kombucha tea.

Step 7: Place the cloth over the opening of the container and secure it with the rubber band. This keeps dust, mold, spores, and vinegar flies out of the fermenting tea.

Step 8: Let the covered container sit undisturbed in a well-ventilated and dark place at a room temperature between 65° and 90°F for 6 to 15 days. To keep the temperature stable, a brew belt is highly recommended (see Resources, page 208).

Step 9: To determine whether the tea is ready, do a taste test every couple of days, starting on the fourth day. The tea should be tart, not sweet. However, it should not be overly sour or vinegary. If the tea is sweet, the sugar hasn't been fully converted. If it tastes like sparkling apple cider, it is ready to drink, unless you want it more tart. If the vinegar taste becomes too prominent, it's probably fermented a bit too long. It won't hurt you to drink at this point, but you won't

FREQUENTLY ASKED QUESTIONS ABOUT KOMBUCHA

My SCOBY sank to the bottom when I made my kombucha. Is it okay?

It is 100 percent okay if your SCOBY sinks. Sink or float—it makes no difference to your kombucha. It won't affect the brew or taste.

My kombucha is still sweet. What did I do wrong?

Your house is probably on the cooler end of the spectrum, and kombucha takes longer to ferment in lower temperatures. Just leave it to ferment longer. I use a brew belt (see Resources, page 208) for a dependable temperature. You can also use a heating pad, but brew belts provide a consistent temperature that is more easily controlled than that of a heating pad.

There is mold on my SCOBY. Is it still safe to consume the tea?

No, it's not safe! Throw the tea and the SCOBY out immediately. As for why this happened, there are a couple of possibilities. Sometimes people do not use the right ratio of sugar and tea to starter culture, and so the tea doesn't ferment properly. Be exact in your measurements. The other cause can be airborne molds in the house. I have had a few people develop this problem because of a leaky roof or by placing their pot in a closet that had poor air circulation.

My tea has a terrible odor. Is it safe to drink?

Your kombucha should have a neutral odor at first, and then gradually take on a more vinegary smell. If you begin to notice a rotten or unpleasant odor, toss the liquid and carefully examine the SCOBY for any signs of mold. If the SCOBY has no mold, simply start again with fresh filtered water and starter tea. If there is mold on the SCOBY, toss everything and start again with all new ingredients.

How long will my SCOBY last?

The SCOBY will last a long time, but not forever. If it turns black or starts to develop mold, it's time to toss it.

Can I cut up my SCOBY?

Yes, absolutely. You only need a part of the SCOBY to ferment the tea. You can even make a pot of kombucha without the SCOBY and just use the starter tea. It will take up to three weeks, but it can be done.

How do I increase the carbonation of my kombucha tea?

One of the reasons your kombucha may not be bubbly is because it's fermented for too long. The bacteria in kombucha eat the sugar, and the yeasts turn the sugar they consume into carbonation. When the bacteria run out of food, the kombucha goes flat. Don't let it get vinegary, and it will stay bubbly.

CHAPTER FOUR

The Wisdom and Magic of Cultured Vegetables

For thousands of years, people preserved their food using the process of lacto-fermentation. They would chop up vegetables, add spices and salt, and submerge the entire mixture under water. They would then wait for a few days for an inexplicable magic to happen. The results were—and still are—some of the most nutritious foods on the planet: cultured vegetables. Placed in a cold environment, these vegetables will last for at least nine months, and the taste will mature with age, taking on wonderful nuanced flavors at different stages, much like a fine wine does. Culturing vegetables is super easy and doesn't require heating, boiling, or hours spent over a hot stove as canning does.

Many of you have probably never heard of *lacto-fermentation*. This type of preservation happens when *Lactobacilli*, a good bacteria found naturally on vegetables, converts the starches and sugars of the vegetables into lactic acid, a natural preservative that inhibits the growth of harmful bacteria. Lactic acid makes the environment surrounding the food too acidic for dangerous bacteria to survive, but keeps the acid at a level in which good bacteria thrive, thus creating a powerful probiotic. Lacto-fermentation also partially digests the food, starting the process of breaking it down into its component parts and making it easier for our bodies to get the most out of it. It also unlocks additional nutrients—

uncultured veggies. The enhanced probiotics, enzymes, and vitamins in cultured vegetables make them powerhouse foods.

Unfortunately, lacto-fermentation is one of the beneficial processes that's been pushed aside in the name of convenience. In an attempt to make foods more shelf stable, the food industry changed the way these foods are created, destroying all that good nutrition in the process. They replaced lacto-fermentation with canning—using a vinegar brine and heat, which kills all the naturally occurring beneficial bacteria and enzymes along with the vitamin C. Because of canning, most people now eat less than optimum versions of foods that were once created through lacto-fermentation. Most sauerkrauts and pickles that you buy at the store simply don't have the amazing health benefits of their homemade counterparts.

But you can start enjoying the advantages of these foods. Some companies have actually moved back to the lacto-fermentation process, plus there's a huge community of people who are interested in culturing their own vegetables. When you're looking for pickles and krauts that have been created using this old-fashioned method, look for products in the refrigerator section of your health-food store and for one that does not contain vinegar. Many of them even say *active cultures* right on the label, so you'll know they're made using lacto-fermentation.

Lacto-fermentation takes ordinary vegetables and makes them even more nutritious by adding vitamins, making the vitamins more bioavailable, and supercharging them with probiotics. Plus the veggies are bubbly, fizzy, and utterly delicious! Lacto-fermentation preserves them, so they can preserve you. I love that these special foods showed up to help me on my life's journey.

The Health Benefits of Cultured Vegetables

Cultured vegetables contain unique bacteria that are unsurpassed as aids to digesting proteins and to repairing the damage done to your gut by processed foods. Dr. Natasha Campbell-McBride, author of *Gut and Psychology Syndrome*, treats many patients with digestive problems, autism, learning disabilities, neurological disorders, psychiatric disorders, and immune disorders. In an interview she did with Dr. Joseph Mercola, an

for the final absorption and digestion of nutrients, water, and electrolytes that come from the foods we eat. Here's what she had to say:

> Our digestive system is lined by very specialized cells, which are called enterocytes. These little cells only live for a few days. They work very hard. They live for two or three days. Then they get too old, too worn out, and the body shuts them off. They die and they get shed off. They get replaced by newly born, healthy baby enterocytes. The cell regeneration process in your gut lining is very, very active. It's a very active process . . .
>
> We have a real chance to heal and seal our damaged gut lining, thanks to this wonderful process of cell regeneration.
>
> But here's the catch: In order for the body to give birth to healthy functioning baby enterocytes, it needs two factors. It needs building blocks for them, because they're made out of certain nutrients. They're made out of proteins, out of certain fats, vitamins, enzymes, and other active molecules. All these building blocks need to be provided for the gut lining to give birth to the cells. That's one. Second, it needs the whole process to be orchestrated by the beneficial microbes in our digestive system, by the beneficial healthy gut flora.[9]

In addition to providing many of the vitamins and minerals necessary to heal the gut, cultured veggies are great at controlling and eliminating a *Candida* imbalance.[10] Having an overabundance of candida causes many of the same symptoms as irritable bowel syndrome (IBS).

When I made cultured veggies a constant companion in my diet, I saw a huge change in my allergies. Spring had been a very painful season for me since my teenage years. I would sneeze. I'd feel blurry. My head and sinuses would ache. All in all, it was just a nasty experience—I would be in misery for weeks on end. But cultured vegetables—with their high doses of vitamin C and their anti-inflammatory properties—greatly reduced my symptoms. When you experience an allergic reaction to something, your body is overreacting to a substance that it should ignore. Your body is treating the substance as a foreign invader, and it creates inflammation to protect itself. This inflammation causes many of the distressing side effects of your allergies. In response to an allergic reaction, your adrenal glands release hormones that bolster your immune system so it can deal with the allergen. To create these hormones, the adrenals need large amounts of vitamins B and C. This hurts you in two ways: it uses up these essential vitamins so they aren't available for other physiological functions, and it uses them up so the adrenals can't do their work. If your adrenals are too fatigued, you will experience worse allergy symptoms. It was just recently—after 40 years of struggle—that I eliminated all my seasonal allergies. It was a combination of cultured foods and other supplements that I added that have allowed me to live a normal life in the spring now.[11]

I've also seen cultured vegetables work wonders on colds and flus. Whenever anyone in my family starts coming down with something, I just grab a spoonful of these veggies. They work like a SWAT team inside your body, fighting off all kinds of viruses and harmful bacteria. They even got me through a bout of food poisoning. Several years ago, Ron, Maci, and I ate some bad artichoke dip that sent us all to bed. As I lay there moaning, I got mad and decided that I wasn't going down without a fight. I dragged myself to the kitchen, ate two big spoonfuls of cultured veggies, and went back to bed. In about a half hour, I was doing dishes. Ron and Maci were almost crying as they asked me how I could be up and about. It was those veggies! They work so fast bringing you back to health that it always astonishes me. And the juice is every bit as powerful as the vegetables. In fact, one of my favorite stories of fighting a flu with veggie juice is about my son, DJ.

DJ was very sick with a stomach flu, and he was in considerable pain because of the stomach cramps. So, being a mother on a mission, I went to his home with pickle juice in hand. When I walked into his darkened bedroom, I found him in sorry shape. He hadn't slept because of his cramps, he wasn't able to keep anything down, and he had a fever. After expressing the proper sympathy, I got down to business. I placed a jar with a half cup of homemade pickle juice on the night table and said, "Just take small sips of this every half hour until the juice is gone. If you do, you'll be up watching TV and eating some rice by tonight." Lo and behold, when I went back later that evening, he was sitting on the sofa watching TV and eating a bowl of plain rice. It made me so happy. DJ is the kindest soul I know, and when he's in pain, it just about kills me.

I've heard so many stories of people finding relief from severe vomiting and stomach distress just a few hours after drinking cultured-vegetable juice that I've lost count. It's the most effective remedy I know for this kind of malady. The fact that this food has such powerful healing properties is becoming common knowledge for everyone who makes and eats cultured vegetables—because they experience it in their own lives. I hope you find the same to be true. I'd love to hear your stories, too!

Making Cultured Vegetables

There are three basic methods used to make cultured vegetables: no culture, with kefir whey, and with Caldwell's Starter Culture. I have my favorite method, but any one of them gets the job done.

No matter the method, you first have to choose a fermenting vessel. You can use a canning jar with a lid, a crock with a lid, a clamp-down lidded jar that has a gasket, or my favorite, a jar with an airlock. Airlock jars create a low-oxygen (anaerobic) environment, in which lactic-acid bacteria thrive. I think this setting produces the best results, and there's less chance of mold developing.

Then decide whether or not you want to use a culture. You can certainly make your vegetables without one, but the good bacteria will stay at a higher level longer if you add a culture. The culture will also increase your body's own ability to use and grow these benefi-cial bacteria inside of you. I've given a quick overview of the three methods below. Once you've figured out which method you want to use, the fermentation process for all three is pretty much the same. You'll find the fermentation procedure after the descriptions of the methods.

Method 1: No Culture

You can make cultured vegetables by simply placing your vegetables in a container and submerging them in water. You must add salt with this method—about 1 teaspoon per 1 quart of vegetables—to inhibit the growth of bad bacteria and to create an environment that is safe. The good bacteria will dominate and keep out harmful pathogens.

Method 2: Kefir Whey

This is a great way to use the kefir whey left over from making Kefir Cheese (see page

BASIC CULTURED VEGETABLES

Step 1: Choose a container large enough to hold the veggies—generally a 1-quart, 2-quart, or 1-gallon vessel—that can be securely sealed.

Step 2: Prepare the Caldwell Starter Culture, if using:

- **For 1 quart:** ¼ packet Caldwell's Starter Culture plus ½ teaspoon sugar or fruit juice mixed with ¼ cup water.

- **For 2 quarts:** ½ packet Caldwell's Starter Culture plus 1 teaspoon sugar or fruit juice mixed with ½ cup water.

- **For 1 gallon:** 1 packet Caldwell's Starter Culture plus 2 teaspoons sugar or fruit juice mixed with 1 cup water.

Step 3: Prepare the vegetables.

Step 4: Pack the vegetables and salt, if using, in the container.

Step 5: Add the culture, if using—prepared Caldwell Starter or Kefir Whey—and fill the container with filtered water, leaving at least 2 inches of headspace at the top to let the vegetables bubble and expand as they ferment.

Step 6: Seal the container and let it sit on your kitchen counter, out of direct sunlight, for 6 days.

Step 7: Check the vegetables every day to make sure they are fully submerged in the water. If they have risen above the water, simply push them down so they are fully covered. If any mold formed because the veggies rose above

like. It's not necessary for safe fermentation as above, but the salt will keep your vegetables crunchy; without it, they will be soft and limp.

Method 3: Caldwell's Starter Culture Packets

This is my favorite method for making cultured vegetables. When I met the people who make these cultures and learned the science behind it, I was impressed. But it was after I used them and saw the results that I was convinced. They told me that quantities of good bacteria stay at a higher level longer with their product. I witnessed this myself when, after a year and a half, I pulled some veggies that I had cultured with this method from the back of my fridge, and they were still bubbly and delicious. Making cultured vegetables with these packets can knock out flus and colds twice as fast as other cultured vegetables I've made. I love them, and I've found that my students have the most success with this method as well.

To make your veggies with a Caldwell's Starter Culture, you simply have to activate the culture by mixing it with water and sugar or fruit or vegeta-

per quart of vegetables. Just mix it all together, and let the mixture sit for 5 to 15 minutes. The sugar will quickly be consumed by the bacteria cultures, so there is no need to worry about the added sugar. Generally, I mix the culture and then prep the vegetables while the culture activates. With this method, salt isn't necessary for safety, but it will keep your veggies crunchy.

You can use the process described in the Basic Cultured Vegetables recipe on page 36 with any of the three methods listed above, but I find that the no-culture method only works well for sauerkrauts. I prefer using a culture. Feel free to play with different vegetables and spices. I've included quite a few recipes for my favorite cultured veggies in Part II of this book. But there are so many people who have created new and inventive flavors that I would hate to have you limit yourself to just these recipes. Once you get the hang of culturing, I'm sure you'll get creative, too.

FREQUENTLY ASKED QUESTIONS ABOUT CULTURED VEGETABLES

Can cultured vegetables develop botulism?

No. Botulism is reserved for canned goods because the heat used in canning kills all the good bacteria. When culturing foods, the healthy bacteria thrive and make it impossible for the bacteria that cause botulism to survive.

How long do I culture my vegetables on the kitchen counter? Can I leave them longer?

For most vegetables, culturing takes six days at room temperature. There are a few vegetables that will culture in only three days, but these shorter times are indicated in the specific recipes in Part II. If you culture the vegetables longer than six days, they can get too yeasty; the flavor will change, and not for the better. However, the veggies still have benefits and are safe to eat. The vegetables will continue to ferment after you place them in the fridge, but at a slower rate. The flavors develop and age like a fine wine!

How long can I store my cultured veggies?

In the refrigerator, cultured veggies will keep for at least nine months, and sometimes longer. They continue to ferment, but at a much slower rate. I find that many of my vegetables taste better after six weeks in the fridge. It's fun to taste your vegetables at different stages to find out when you like them best.

Can these foods be stored out of the fridge after they have been fermented?

Technically, cultured vegetables can be stored in a cooler basement or cold cellar. However, they will continue to ferment and in short order, they won't taste very good. Cultured veggies do best and taste best at the colder temperatures of a refrigerator.

How will I know if my vegetables are properly fermented?

They will taste sour and the liquid they are in will look bubbly. If your culturing has gone wrong, you will know this by the strong, unappetizing odor the veggies will give off.

What are the white spots on my veggies?

This is harmless mold. If the vegetables rise up above the water level, they will develop mold. Simply scoop out the moldy vegetables and resubmerge the rest under the water. Check from time to time while they are fermenting to make sure they remain submerged.

CHAPTER FIVE

Sprouted Grains and Sourdough: The Answer to So Many Problems

The last items I am going to discuss are sprouted grains and sourdough bread. Unlike the other foods we've covered, these aren't necessarily living probiotic foods. The good bacteria (*Lactobacilli*) transform the bread through fermentation prior to baking. The heat kills the beneficial bacteria, but the fermentation process has already developed many vitamins and minerals that aren't found in regular grain. So these grains are supercharged, plus the fermentation process alters the structure of the grains so that they're more easily digested.

As part of my fermented food journey, I discovered that grains are not the same as they once were. For thousands of years, sheaths of grain would be cut by hand, stacked in the fields, and left to be gathered the next day. The morning dew would cause the grains to sprout, thereby unlocking the nutrients and deactivating the phytic acid and enzyme inhibitors, making the grains easy to digest. Then the workers would gather the grains and take the seeds off the stalks to be used. Today we have combines that remove the seeds instantly, never allowing the grains to sprout.

flour in the same way that sprouting does—releasing nutrients and creating a more digestible product. This process doesn't use sprouted flour, but bread made this way has the same benefits as bread made with sprouted flour. But this transformation is dependent on letting the dough culture for many hours at room temperature. It takes at least seven hours for these dramatic changes to occur. Now with instant yeasts, the bread rises so quickly that it never has a chance to be transformed.

What does this mean for us? In my life, it meant painful days of irritable bowel syndrome (IBS) for my daughter Maci. And for thousands of others, it means a gluten-free diet. However, now there are other options.

You can buy sprouted flour and sprouted bread products at any health-food store. But I prefer to bake homemade sourdough and sprouted breads and to make my own flours, because I can control how the products are created. I know that the grains have sprouted just right and that my sourdough bread has risen long enough.

Making your own sprouted flour takes some equipment, but it's definitely worth the investment. I sprout 14 pounds of flour at a time, and I use it in nearly all of my baking. It has been life changing for my family and me.

Ancient cultures knew the benefits of soaking and sprouting grains because they experienced them firsthand. They passed these cultures down through generations like heirlooms. And until fairly recently, sourdough starters bubbling on kitchen counters were the norm and not the exception. My belief is that these traditional techniques carry much wisdom that we need today. In an era when fast breads are wreaking havoc on our guts, sourdough and sprouted grains can be the answer for so many people dealing with problems concerning grains.

Health Benefits of Sprouted Grains and Sourdough

While many of us struggle to digest grains, we flourish when these same grains are sprouted. The process of sprouting improves the quality of the grain, making it more nutrient dense. These grains provide us with vitamins and minerals that affect every aspect of our well-being—from mood to digestion to immunity. Sally Fallon, president of the Weston Price Foundation and the author of *Nourishing Traditions*, sums up the benefits of sprout-

The process of germination not only produces vitamin C but also changes the composition of the grain and seeds in numerous beneficial ways. Sprouting increases vitamin B content, especially B2, B5, and B6, and carotene increases dramatically—sometimes eightfold. Even more important, sprouting neutralizes phytic acid, a substance present in the bran of all grains that inhibits absorption of calcium, magnesium, iron, copper and zinc; sprouting also reduces enzyme inhibitors present in all seeds.[12]

One of the other wonderful advantages of sprouted grains is that they are considered low glycemic. Sprouting the grain returns it to a plant state. This allows sprouted grains to digest as vegetables in the body. Without sprouting, grains digest as starches.[13] What does this mean for you? Basically, vegetables are much easier to break down than starches, which use pancreatic enzymes. Most people don't produce these enzymes in large quantities, so an overabundance of starches taxes the pancreas. If you are diabetic, this is not good.

But here's something everyone will love: Sprouting grains increases their satiety factor—meaning they fill you up faster, which is great for weight management. I actually had a woman at our co-op come up to me and tell me how she began losing weight when she started making sprouted flour and baking her own sprouted breads. And a few notes I've received from others with similar outcomes show that her experience isn't unique.

Like sprouted grains, when you use a sourdough starter to make bread, mineral inhibitors are deactivated and the bioavailability of nutrients increases. While the sprouting of grains happens with water, the transformation of sourdough to a healthier form that is easier to digest is due to good bacteria working with yeast in symbiosis. This action also makes the bread resistant to mold and staleness.

Making Sprouted White-Wheat Flour

I love using sprouted grains for baking—especially bread. And luckily, the process of making sprouted flour is really simple; however, you do need a dehydrator and a grain mill before you begin. Check out the Resources (page 208) for more information on this equipment. When soaking wheat berries, or any grain, do not oversprout them. The tails should be very tiny; you should have to look closely to see them. This is the perfect degree of

In the recipe below, you'll be making white-wheat flour, but you can use this process to make flour from any grains. So choose what you like: whole wheat, rye, spelt, kamut, barley—they're all delicious. In the recipes in this book, I always list this sprouted white-wheat flour, but feel free to substitute any sprouted flour.

You can use this flour just like you would any all-purpose flour in any recipe. And depending on how often you bake, the flour could last you for a while. I go through it pretty quickly, but it will keep for six months when stored at room temperature, or longer in the refrigerator.

SOURDOUGH BREAD

Sourdough bread is hands down my favorite cultured food to make—I love taking a warm loaf from the oven. See Donna's Sourdough Bread on page 129; I guarantee you'll love it, and so will your body.

To make sourdough bread, you'll need a starter culture. I purchased mine, and I recommend this over making your own starter. It takes years to develop a well-flavored sourdough that works successfully to rise your bread. It will last you a lifetime if you take care of it. You will also be able to share the starter with friends and family, so they can bake sourdough bread, too. To find a good starter culture, refer to the Resources on page 208.

Remember that once you have the starter culture, you will have to care for it and feed it with flour and water on a regular basis. The starter you get should come with instructions for its care and feeding, but I've also outlined some basics, including some troubleshooting, at www.culturedfoodlife.com/how-to-care-for-your-sourdough-starter, just in case you want or need more information. I know it may seem like a lot of work, but don't worry, it's hard to kill a sourdough starter. Even after the grossest neglect,

SPROUTED WHITE-WHEAT FLOUR

Makes 14¼ cups sprouted flour

5 pounds white wheat berries

....

Step 1: Place the grains in a large glass bowl, and add enough filtered water to cover the grain by at least 1 inch.

Step 2: Let the bowl sit for 36 hours. The grains will sprout tiny little tails, and the water will be a bit bubbly.

FREQUENTLY ASKED QUESTIONS ABOUT SPROUTED GRAINS AND SOURDOUGH

How long should I let my grains sprout?

The optimal amount of time to sprout your grains is 36 hours. You will see very tiny white stubs coming out of the ends of the grains. Long sprouts on the grains are not desirable. A tiny sprout is best. When you sprout it longer, it alters the grain, reducing its beneficial properties.

Is there gluten in sprouted flour? Can I eat it if I'm gluten sensitive?

The grain is completely transformed when it is sprouted. Many who struggle with regular grains do great on sprouted grains, as this is an entirely new food. It digests like a vegetable rather than a grain. If you are gluten intolerant, it is a sign that your digestive system and its eco-world are not working properly, and sometimes even sprouted grains cannot be tolerated. It depends on the degree of damage that your gut has sustained. Many people do fine on sprouted grains, but if you feel you do not, then I recommend first adding other cultured foods to your diet at every meal to heal your gut. With some time, you'll be able to enjoy sprouted or sourdough breads.

How long does sprouted flour keep after milling?

Sprouted flour can be stored at room temperature for six months after milling, unlike unsprouted flour, which must be used immediately so it doesn't go rancid. The germ cell of the grain is the part that degrades and becomes rancid when milled. When grains are sprouted, the germ cell is consumed by the endosperm and it is no longer in a state that can become rancid. This is one of the many advantages of sprouted flour.

Can I use sprouted flour as a substitute for regular flour?

Yes, you can substitute sprouted flour for conventional flour one-to-one in most recipes. I do this all the time, and it works great.

Are the bacteria in sourdough bread killed when you bake the bread?

Yes, anytime you heat bacteria you kill them. However, the transformation of the bread has already taken place during the rising phase. The bacteria unlock the nutrients, and the vitamins and minerals become more accessible.

My starter is bubbly but not rising. Can I use it?

Your starter must be rising in the jar, as this is how you'll know it's ready to use. If it is just bubbly but not rising, you need to feed it until it starts to rise in the jar. Then it's ready to rise your bread. Check out my website for more info: www.culturedfoodlife.com/how-to-care-for-your-sourdough-starter.

Why is my bread taking forever to rise?

It's most likely that your sourdough starter is not active enough. Temperature can also slow down the rising process, but most likely, your starter was sluggish and not fed enough. Let the starter sit on the counter and see if it will rise. It may just take longer, but if it does not rise, then your starter needs to be revived.

What is the brown liquid on top of my starter?

This is called the *hooch*, and it's the sign of a starving sourdough starter. It needs to be fed, because it has consumed all the nutrients in the flour. Pour off this liquid and replace it with water, or just mix the hooch back into the starter; then add fresh flour and more water because your starter is hungry.

How often should I feed my sourdough starter?

If you are storing your sourdough starter in the refrigerator, you should feed it at least once a week. If you forget to feed it, take it out of the fridge and feed it once in the morning and once at night for three days to revive it. It should then be strong and ready to use again to rise your bread.

PART II

Recipes with Cultured Foods

CHAPTER SIX

Breakfast Treats and Smoothies

BREAKFAST TREATS

Breakfast is my favorite meal of the day, which is why I often have it for lunch, too. It's easy and quick, and it fills me up, especially when it's loaded with kefir. I was reminded of the filling power of kefir when I went to New York for a weekend and didn't have the option of kefir for breakfast. I missed it terribly, and I thought about food a lot more than normal because I didn't feel nearly as nourished and satisfied as usual. Kefir really does make me feel good. It does just what food should do—it helps me from the inside out. Kefir and cultured foods make me shine. And now you can start your day with some kefir, too!

HERBED OMELET WITH KEFIR HOLLANDAISE SAUCE

My daughter Holli has a wonderful friend who was allergic to eggs, but after introducing her and her family to cultured foods, she can now eat them. Not only that—she also raises and cares for her own chicken! Its fresh eggs were the inspiration for this omelet.

Makes 2 servings

1 heaping tablespoon grated Parmesan cheese

1 garlic clove, minced

2 teaspoons minced fresh rosemary

2 teaspoons minced parsley

1 tablespoon olive oil

4 large eggs

2 tablespoons milk

Celtic Sea Salt to taste

White pepper to taste

¼ cup shredded pepper Jack cheese

Kefir Hollandaise Sauce (page 188)

....

Mix together the Parmesan cheese, garlic, rosemary, and parsley in a cup and set aside.

Heat a medium skillet over medium-low heat. Add the olive oil and swirl to coat the pan.

Crack the eggs into a bowl and stir in the milk, salt, and white pepper, then grab your whisk and whisk like crazy. You're going to beat as much air as possible into the eggs.

When the oil in the pan is hot enough to make a drop of water hiss, pour in the egg mixture. Don't stir! Let the eggs cook until the bottom starts to set, approximately 1 minute.

Sprinkle the herb mixture and the pepper Jack cheese evenly over the top of the eggs.

With a heat-resistant rubber spatula, gently lift one edge of the eggs toward the center of the pan, while tilting the pan to allow the liquid eggs to flow underneath. Repeat around the edge of the omelet until there's no uncooked egg remaining.

With your spatula, lift one half of the omelet and fold it across and over the other half, lining up the edges. Cook just for another minute or so, flipping the omelet over after 30 seconds, but don't overcook or allow the omelet to turn brown.

SPROUTED GINGER SCONES WITH PEACHES AND KEFIR CREAM

It was late one night and my daughter Maci sent me some pictures of kefir grains for my blog. I felt such love and appreciation for these special microbes that perform for me night and day and never charge me a penny that I teared up as I looked at this picture. I really don't care anymore what others think. I love these little guys; they changed my life and make me happy and healthy. And I think everybody needs to know.

Makes 8 servings

2 cups Sprouted White-Wheat Flour (page 42)

½ cup Sucanat or honey

3 teaspoons baking powder

¼ teaspoon Celtic Sea Salt

6 tablespoons chilled butter, cut into pieces

1 large egg

⅔ cups Basic Kefir (page 15)

1 teaspoon Vanilla Extract (page 204)

¼ cup crystallized ginger

3 large peaches, sliced

1 cup Kefir Whipped Cream (page 183)

....

Preheat the oven to 350°F. Grease baking sheet.

Combine the flour, Sucanat, baking powder, and salt in a large bowl.

Cut in the butter with a pastry blender or two knives used scissor-fashion until mixture looks like large crumbs. (You can also use a food processor; pulse until large crumbs form.)

Combine the egg, kefir, and vanilla in a small bowl, and stir thoroughly to combine.

Stir the wet ingredients into the dry ingredients just until combined. Do not overmix.

Gently stir in the ginger.

If you have a scone pan (one of those neat pans with ready-made divisions), you can just scoop the dough into the pan and bake as directed. If making the scones by hand, turn the dough onto a floured surface and knead four to five times with floured hands. Pat out to ½-inch thickness and cut the dough circles using a biscuit cutter or the rim of a round drinking glass. Place on the prepared

STRAWBERRY SCONES WITH LEMON PROBIOTIC TOPPING

My daughter Maci had a sleepover for her girlfriends, and I made these for breakfast the next morning. They were a hit and have become one of my family's favorites—they're even better the next day. The strawberries make for supermoist scones, and the lemon topping enhances the taste of the strawberries.

Makes 8 servings

For the scones

2 cups Sprouted White-Wheat Flour (page 42)

⅓ cup plus 2 tablespoons Sucanat

2 teaspoons baking powder

¼ teaspoon Celtic Sea Salt

⅓ cup chilled butter, cut into pieces

1 egg

⅔ cup heavy whipping cream

1 teaspoon Vanilla Extract (page 204)

1 cup chopped fresh strawberries

1 egg and 1 teaspoon water, beaten, for the egg wash

2 tablespoons sliced almonds

....

For the lemon probiotic topping

16 ounces full-fat Greek yogurt

¼ cup lemon juice

Zest of 1 lemon

1 tablespoon Basic Kefir (page 15)

2 teaspoons honey or Sucanat, or 2 packets stevia

....

For the scones

Cut in the butter with a pastry blender or two knives used scissor-fashion.

Stir together the egg, cream, and vanilla.

Stir the wet ingredients into the dry, stirring just until moistened.

Fold in the strawberries. The mixture will be very sticky.

If you have a scone pan (one of those neat pans with ready-made divisions) you can just scoop the dough into the pan and bake as directed. If making the scones by hand, turn the dough onto a floured surface and knead four to five times with floured hands. Pat the dough out to ½-inch thickness and cut into circles with a biscuit cutter or the rim of a round drinking glass. Reroll the dough scraps as necessary to make 8 scones. Brush the tops with the egg wash, and sprinkle with remaining 2 tablespoons Sucanat and sliced almonds. Place on the prepared baking sheet.

Bake the scones for 25 to 30 minutes, or until golden brown. Transfer to a wire rack to cool.

To serve the scones, dollop each with a generous spoonful of the lemon topping.

For the lemon probiotic topping

Mix together all the ingredients in a small bowl. (If you're not serving the scones right away, cover and refrigerate the topping until you're ready to use.)

CHOCOLATE KEFIR SOURDOUGH WAFFLES

I was making these waffles one morning when I opened the door for a UPS delivery. As the aroma of chocolate and waffle batter wafted out the door, the deliveryman exclaimed, "What are you making? It smells like Willy Wonka's chocolate factory!" Many months later he delivered the first copies of my self-published book and asked if the waffle recipe was included. I shook my head, and he started to carry my boxes back to the truck, saying the book was incomplete without it. So I put the waffles in this one just for him.

A note before you begin: Levain is a leavening agent that is sometimes called wild yeast. You'll need to make this at least eight hours before you start the waffles. You can make it the night before and leave it covered on your kitchen counter.

Makes 7 servings

For the levain

4 ounces sourdough starter

1 cup whole-wheat flour (not sprouted)

1 cup Basic Kefir (page 15)

....

For the waffle batter

½ cup Dutch-process cocoa

1 teaspoon baking soda

½ teaspoon Celtic Sea Salt

Pinch of cinnamon

2 large eggs

4 tablespoons melted butter

½ cup Sucanat or 4 packets stevia

2 teaspoons Vanilla Extract (page 204)

½ to ¾ cup 65% cacao chocolate chips or dark chocolate chips
(mini chips work especially well)

....

For the levain

Place sourdough starter into a large bowl.

Stir in the flour and kefir and mix thoroughly until combined. The mixture will be quite thick.

Cover the bowl with plastic wrap and set aside on the kitchen counter for at least 8 hours.

For the waffle batter

Stir together the cocoa, baking soda, salt, and cinnamon in a small bowl.

In a separate bowl, whisk the eggs with the melted butter, Sucanat, and vanilla.

Add the cocoa mixture, and stir to combine.

Add the cocoa-and-egg mixture to the levain and stir thoroughly, until there are no streaks of unmixed sourdough in the batter. The batter will start to rise from the baking soda acting with the kefir and sourdough.

Stir in the chocolate chips.

Preheat your waffle iron and cook the waffles according to the manufacturer's instructions. My waffles take 3 to 5 minutes. The waffles will feel soft coming out of the waffle iron, but will crisp up after you remove them.

BANANA BREAD FRENCH TOAST

I always pull out all the stops when my mom visits. I try to think of recipes that will make her ooh and aah, and this was her favorite from a recent visit. It's a love thing: I still want to receive praise from my mom and make her happy. She loves my food like she loves me—with her whole heart.

Makes 5 servings

2 eggs

⅔ cup milk

1 teaspoon Vanilla Extract (page 204; optional)

¼ teaspoon ground cinnamon (optional)

¼ teaspoon ground nutmeg (optional)

Sprouted Banana Bread (page 139)

Maple syrup to serve

....

Beat together the eggs, milk, vanilla, cinnamon, and nutmeg, if using, in a wide flat bowl.

Cut one loaf of Sprouted Banana Bread into 10 slices.

Heat a lightly oiled griddle or skillet over medium-high heat.

Dunk each slice of bread into the egg mixture, soaking both sides.

Place the bread on the griddle and cook each side until golden, approximately 2 to 3 minutes per side.

Serve hot with maple syrup.

KEFIR BREAKFAST PUDDING

When I was a little girl, I pretended we had elves in our house. I imagined they worked for us while we slept, and in the morning we would find a new pair of shoes and breakfast waiting for us. Alas, every morning it was just my mother in the kitchen. There were no shoes. There was no special elfish breakfast. This recipe is like having elves. Just place the ingredients in the fridge the night before, and the next morning you have a thick creamy kefir breakfast pudding . . . just like elves would make!

Makes 1 serving

1 cup Basic Kefir (page 15)

½ cup fruit of your choice, plus extra for topping

¼ cup oatmeal of your choice (old fashioned, rolled, instant, or steel cut)

1½ teaspoons chia seeds

Honey, Sucanat, or stevia to taste (optional)

Place all the ingredients except sweetener in a 1-pint canning jar.

Cap the jar and shake vigorously.

Place the jar in the refrigerator overnight.

When ready to serve, transfer the pudding to a bowl and top it with more fruit and sweetener, if using.

BLUEBERRY KEFIR PUDDING WITH BASIL AND SOAKED ALMONDS

I love this blueberry pudding. The tang of the basil with the tartness of the blueberry kefir is a taste sensation, and the soaked almonds help fill you up with all their good fats. Plus the huge amount of vitamin C and the oodles of good bacteria in it help boost the immune system. This is a great way to start off your day!

Makes 1 serving

1 cup fresh or frozen blueberries

1 cup Basic Kefir (page 15)

2 tablespoons honey or 2 packets stevia

Soaked Salted Almonds (page 85) for garnish

Fresh torn basil for garnish

Place the blueberries, kefir, and sweetener in a blender, and blend on high until smooth.

Transfer the mixture to a bowl, and top with almonds and basil.

BAKED APPLES WITH KEFIR TOPPING

In the winter, sometimes the last thing you want is a cold smoothie. This recipe is a way to eat your kefir and still feel cozy on a frigid morning. It's a warm and comforting breakfast, snack, or dessert. Best of all, it makes the house smell heavenly. You'll be surprised how delicious this tastes!

Makes 2 servings

For the baked apples

2 medium apples (Golden Delicious or Rome Beauty)

2 tablespoons butter

2 tablespoons chopped walnuts

1 tablespoon Sucanat

1 teaspoon ground cinnamon

For the kefir topping

2 cups Basic Kefir (page 15)

4 tablespoons maple syrup or 4 packets stevia

2 teaspoons ground cinnamon

Golden raisins and chopped walnuts for serving (optional)

For the baked apples

Preheat oven to 375°F.

Wash and core the apples almost to the bottom. (Don't cut all the way through.) Peel off a thin strip around the top of the apple. Place the apples in a small baking dish.

Combine the butter, walnuts, Sucanat, and cinnamon in a cup. Fill the cavity of each apple with the mixture, dividing it evenly between the two apples.

Pour ¼ cup of water into the bottom of the baking dish. Bake for 30 minutes.

For the kefir topping

JANE'S KEFIR COTTAGE CHEESE

Jane and her husband run the local farm where I buy my milk for kefir. Everyone raves about Jane's kefir cottage cheese—they sell a lot of it each week. And those of us who know her aren't surprised that she has come up with such a delicious recipe: She puts her heart into everything she does. You'll be hard pressed to find any cottage cheese out there that is better for you. I top it with a little milk to make it creamy, and I like it with a chopped baked apple on top. I also use this recipe to make dip at least three times a week—see Apple Kefir Cottage Cheese (page 59), Blueberry Kefir Cottage Cheese (page 60), and Tuscan Kefir Cottage Cheese Dip (page 76). I'm thankful to Jane not only for coming up with this recipe but also for graciously allowing me to use it in this book.

A note before you begin: The amount of kefir you use when making this recipe is up to you. The more you use, the quicker the cheese sets. I generally go toward the higher quantity and use 2 cups of kefir. Also, keep in mind that a thermometer is a requirement for this recipe. You need to keep the temperature consistent so you don't kill the beneficial bacteria. You can use a standard candy or meat thermometer; these generally have temperatures that range from 32° to 225°F (0 to 100° C).

Makes 4 to 5 servings

1 gallon raw or pasteurized milk

1 to 2 cups Basic Kefir (page 15)

¼ to ½ teaspoon Celtic Sea Salt (optional)

Cream or milk for serving (optional)

....

Pour the milk into a large pot and add the kefir.

Heat the mixture to 80°F and turn off the heat; then cover the pot and let the mixture sit for 24 hours, or until thickened. A thick curd will form. The curd shrinks away from the sides of the pan a bit, and you may see a thin layer of whey on the top. You may even notice some cracks forming on the surface.

After 24 hours, slowly bring the mixture to 100°F over low heat, stirring every few minutes to break up the curds on the bottom of the pan so they don't burn. You will know when the cottage cheese is done when the whey separates from the curd. The whey is a clear yellowish liquid. This process takes approximately 20 minutes.

Place a strainer lined with cheesecloth over a large bowl and pour the curds and whey in.

Gather up the sides of the cheesecloth and twist, so that the whey drains through the cheesecloth. The finished curds may have combined somewhat, but they're easy to separate.

APPLE KEFIR COTTAGE CHEESE

Jane's Kefir Cottage Cheese is always in my fridge. I like it plain, with a little cream added, or with fruit, as offered here. Use your imagination and taste buds to develop your own delicious combinations.

Makes 1 serving

1 cup Jane's Kefir Cottage Cheese (page 58)

1 apple, chopped

¼ cup chopped walnuts

2 tablespoons honey or 2 packets stevia

Liberal pinch of cinnamon

....

Combine all the ingredients in a small bowl and mix thoroughly.

BLUEBERRY KEFIR COTTAGE CHEESE

I can't tell you how many times I eat this during the week. I usually have it for breakfast, but more and more, I have it for lunch, because it is fast, easy, and filling. This dish takes five minutes for me to spoon into a bowl. Who says fast food can't be good for you!

Makes 1 serving

1 cup Jane's Kefir Cottage Cheese (page 58)

¾ cup fresh or frozen (thawed) blueberries

2 tablespoons honey or 2 packets stevia

1 tablespoon sliced almonds

1 teaspoon dried cranberries or goji berries

Liberal pinch of cinnamon

Combine all the ingredients in a small bowl and mix thoroughly.

SMOOTHIES

Smoothies are the most common way to enjoy kefir, and they are a great breakfast option. They are also the easiest way to get your kids to enjoy the benefits of kefir. These delicious treats are loaded with calcium, magnesium, the B vitamins, vitamin C, and lots of probiotics—plus, they fill you up and stave off hunger for hours. Kefir smoothies are my secret weapons for staying healthy and happy.

BASIC KEFIR FRUIT SMOOTHIE

One Saturday at the lake where we spend our weekends, someone had gotten a fruit smoothie from a fast-food chain. We compared ingredients. Their yogurt smoothie had 22 ingredients and my kefir smoothie had 4. I bet you know which one tasted better.

A note before you begin: Bananas, blueberries, strawberries, peaches, oranges, and mangoes all work well in smoothies. If you like frothy and bubbly smoothies, add ½ cup of ice to this or any of the smoothie recipes.

Makes 1 serving

1 cup Basic Kefir (page 15)

1 cup fresh or frozen fruit of your choice

Honey, Sucanat, or stevia to taste

½ cup ice (optional)

....

Place all the ingredients in a blender and mix at high speed until smooth. Serve immediately.

PLUM AND BANANA KEFIR SMOOTHIE

This summer I became addicted to plums. I like the really dark purple ones with the red flesh (called black plums) that taste like candy. I paired one with a banana in a smoothie, and it was supercreamy and the prettiest lilac color. I hope you enjoy this smoothie as much as I do. And remember, when shopping for plums, the more color it has, the more antioxidants it contains and the better it is for you.

Makes 1 serving

1 cup Basic Kefir (page 15)

1 black plum

1 banana

Honey, Sucanat, or stevia to taste

Kefir Whipped Cream (page 183) for serving

Chopped cacao nibs for serving

Place all the ingredients in a blender and mix at high speed until smooth.

Pour the smoothie into a glass and top with the whipped cream and cacao nibs. Serve immediately.

PURPLE COW KEFIR SMOOTHIE

You can make this with green grapes instead of purple. It will be more tangy than sweet, but it will be equally good. You could call it a green cow smoothie, but a Kermit smoothie sounds like much more fun.

A note before you begin: Freeze the grapes for a frosty drink.

Makes 1 serving

1 cup purple grapes

½ cup Kefir Cheese (page 17)

½ cup Basic Kefir (page 15)

Honey, Sucanat, or stevia to taste

Place all the ingredients in a blender and mix at high speed until smooth. Serve immediately.

PEACH-CARROT KEFIR SMOOTHIE

I love it when my food looks pretty. The carrots and slices of ginger added to the fresh peaches in this smoothie paint a great picture. Come on . . . play with your food!

Makes 1 serving

1 cup Basic Kefir (page 15)

1 cup frozen peaches

1 carrot, chopped

3 strawberries, tops included

½-inch slice fresh ginger, peeled

Honey, Sucanat, or stevia to taste

. . . .

Place all the ingredients in a blender and mix at high speed until smooth. Serve immediately.

BLUE CACAO KEFIR SMOOTHIE

I use blackberries in kefir smoothies throughout the summer because I have a blackberry bush in my backyard. If you've never combined blackberries and cacao powder before, believe me, you're in for a treat! And if you're feeling extra decadent, top this with a little fresh Kefir Whipped Cream (page 183) and a few cacao nibs.

Makes 1 serving

½ cup Kefir Cheese (page 17)

½ cup Basic Kefir (page 15)

½ cup frozen blackberries

⅓ cup fresh parsley

3 whole strawberries, tops included

1 tablespoon cacao powder or cocoa powder

Honey, Sucanat, or stevia to taste (optional)

Place all the ingredients in a blender and mix at high speed until smooth. Serve immediately.

COCONUT-MANGO KEFIR SMOOTHIE

When I was in the Caribbean I had a drink that wowed me. I talked to the waiter about it, and he said in his Jamaican accent, "Mum, it is coconut milk and mango. That is the secret." As soon as I got home, I devised this recipe and have been enjoying it ever since. It tastes best if you hum a little reggae when you blend it.

A note before you begin: To save time, buy chopped mango from the produce or freezer aisles of your supermarket.

Makes 4 servings

3 mangoes, peeled, pitted, and chopped (about 4 cups)

14 ounces coconut milk

1 cup Basic Kefir (page 15)

1 cup ice

¼ cup honey

Pinch of salt

Mint sprigs for serving (optional)

Place all the ingredients in a blender and mix at high speed until very smooth, about 2 to 3 minutes, scraping down sides as necessary.

Divide the smoothie between four glasses, and garnish with mint, if desired.

CHAPTER SEVEN

Dips and Appetizers

DIPS

Dips are a great way to introduce friends and family to just how tasty cultured foods can be. Because kefir is so versatile, it's an amazing healthy base for many different flavors. These dips are what I bring most often to parties, and people never know they're eating healthy probiotics until I tell them.

APPLE, KEFIR, AND BLUE CHEESE DIP

I was asked to be on a local TV station to talk about my book, and I served this dip with apple slices. When I was packing up to leave, one of the producers asked if I could leave the dip. He loved the apples and blue cheese combo, and said it was like Roquefort and pears—only better! This is also delicious with crackers or vegetables; don't limit yourself to apples.

A note before you begin: For the best texture, make sure your kefir cheese has drained for 24 hours before making this dip. If you want to experiment, you can substitute Cheddar cheese for the blue cheese, and the dip will be equally delicious; just use a little less lemon juice.

Makes 4 servings

1 cup Kefir Cheese (page 17)

1 cup chopped walnuts or pecans

½ cup crumbled blue cheese

1 small apple, chopped into tiny pieces

3 tablespoons minced pitted dates

Zest and juice of ½ lemon

1½ teaspoons garlic powder

1½ teaspoons onion salt

¼ teaspoon Celtic Sea Salt

¼ cup minced fresh parsley for serving

Add the kefir cheese, walnuts, blue cheese, apple, dates, lemon zest and juice, garlic powder, onion salt, and salt to the work bowl of a food processor, and pulse to mix well.

Place the mixture in a serving dish; cover and refrigerate for at least 1 hour.

Top with parsley before serving.

Storage note: This dip can stored in a covered airtight container in the refrigerator for up to one month.

GARLIC-KEFIR CHEESE DIP

This flavorful dip is a real hit with garlic lovers. Roasting garlic brings out its sweet and nutty flavor. It's much milder than when used raw, so don't be afraid to add the whole head of garlic. If you find an olive oil flavored with basil or other Italian herbs, do go ahead and use it here. This dip is best served with crackers or vegetables.

Makes 8 servings

1 garlic head

¾ cup Kefir Cheese (page 17)

¾ cup grated Pecorino-Romano or Parmesan-Reggiano cheese

3 ounces cream cheese

3 tablespoons olive oil, plus more for serving

Preheat the oven to 375°F.

Slice the top off the garlic head to expose the tops of the individual cloves. Wrap the garlic head in foil and roast it for 1 hour. When the garlic has cooled, separate the cloves and squeeze the garlic out. It will be very soft and will pop right out of the skin.

Place the garlic, cheeses, and olive oil in the work bowl of a food processor. Process until smooth, about 1 minute.

Transfer the dip into a serving bowl and drizzle with a little more olive oil.

Storage note: This dip can be kept in a covered airtight container in the refrigerator for up to one month.

PROBIOTIC GUACAMOLE

This guacamole will last much longer than other guacamoles without turning brown because of the good bacteria and enzymes. If these cultures help prolong the color and life of the food, doesn't it make sense that it will also do the same for you? Remember, wear gloves when seeding and chopping the chile, and avoid touching your face, especially near your eyes.

Makes 6 servings

1 large avocado, scooped out and chopped

⅓ cup Kefir Cheese (page 17)

One small handful cilantro, chopped

½ small serrano chile, chopped

1 teaspoon Celtic Sea Salt

¼ lime

....

Pulse the avocado, kefir cheese, cilantro, serrano chile, and salt in the work bowl of a food processor until mixed, or mix by hand with a fork, mashing the avocado.

Squeeze lime over the guacamole, and pulse or mix again.

Storage note: This dip can be kept in a covered airtight container in the refrigerator for up to three weeks.

CULTURED BEAN DIP

I made this recipe for a Super Bowl party, and as I watched my son eat this dip with sprouted corn chips, I started counting in my head all the friendly bacteria he had just consumed. I'm probably the only person I know who lies in bed at night and tries to remember the names of all the bacteria and yeast in kefir. Forget football—these are my sports stats! For an extra bang, add a layer of Probiotic Guacamole (page 70) between the beans and the cheese.

Makes 12 servings

1½ cups of refried pinto beans

1 cup Kefir Cheese (page 17)

2 tablespoons taco seasoning

1 cup Cultured Border Salsa (page 77)

1 cup of shredded Monterey Jack cheese

½ cup chopped black olives

½ cup chopped green onions

. . . .

Spread the refried beans in an 8-inch square baking dish.

Mix together the kefir cheese and the taco seasoning, and spread the mixture over the beans.

Layer the salsa on top of the kefir cheese; then add the layer of Monterey Jack cheese.

Sprinkle the olives and green onions over the dip.

Storage note: This dip can be kept in a covered airtight container in the refrigerator for up to two weeks.

FERMENTED HUMMUS

Hummus is already considered a healthy food, and fermenting it makes it even more nutritious by increasing the availability of the vitamin content and adding probiotics. This hummus becomes pre-digested, so the body has no trouble assimilating it. This creates less stress on the body. Like any cultured food, it becomes supercharged, giving you more energy for your day.

Makes 10 servings

1 pound garbanzo beans, preferably soaked and sprouted

3 cloves Fermented Garlic (page 201)

6 tablespoons olive oil

4 tablespoons lemon juice

2 to 3 tablespoons raw tahini

¼ teaspoon Celtic Sea Salt

1 teaspoon cumin (optional)

1 teaspoon hot curry powder (optional)

1 teaspoon red pepper flakes or Aleppo pepper (optional)

....

Place the beans, garlic, olive oil, and lemon juice in a food processor or blender, and pulse until smooth.

Add the tahini and salt, along with the cumin, curry powder, and red pepper flakes, if using. Pulse until the hummus is smooth (add more olive oil, if necessary).

Storage note: The hummus can be kept in a covered airtight container in the refrigerator for up to three weeks.

CULTURED GRINGO DIP

This dip is a hit at my cultured food classes. People love it, and after class they always ask if there's any left. It's a powerhouse dish with two cultured veggies plus kefir cheese. There are more probiotics in this dish than most people get in months. Eat it with sprouted corn chips for even more benefits!

Makes 4 servings

2 medium avocados

1 cup Kefir Cheese (page 17) or sour cream

5 Fermented Cherry Tomatoes That Pop (page 116)

6 to 7 slices Fermented Jalapeños (page 202), or more if you like it hotter

....

Scoop the avocado flesh into the work bowl of a food processor.

Add the kefir cheese, tomatoes, and jalapeños, and pulse until well combined.

Storage note: This dip can be kept in a covered airtight container in the refrigerator for up to one month.

KEFIR ONION DIP

This is a dip I make every year for the Super Bowl. My husband loves French Onion dip, but store-bought onion dips give him terrible indigestion. So now I make it at home, and he loves it so much that I hardly get a bite—but no more indigestion. You can serve this dip with any kind of chips, but I make my own by thinly slicing potatoes and frying them in peanut oil until they're brown and crispy.

A note before you begin: I like to use homemade kefir cheese, but if you don't have time to make it, The Greek Gods brand kefir cheese, available in health and natural food stores, is a good substitute.

Makes 6 servings

1 tablespoon butter or olive oil

1 medium or large onion, finely chopped

1 large leek, finely chopped (optional)

1½ cups Kefir Cheese (page 17)

Juice of 1 small lemon

1 teaspoon Celtic Sea Salt

1 teaspoon paprika

Poppy seeds for serving (optional)

Sesame seeds for serving (optional)

Dehydrated onions for serving (optional)

....

Melt the butter in a medium skillet over medium-high heat.

Add the onion and leek, if using, and cook until softened, about 5 to 7 minutes. Let cool until just warm.

Transfer the onion mixture to a food processor. Add the cheese, lemon juice, salt, and paprika. Pulse several times until the mixture is well combined and smooth.

Transfer the dip to a serving bowl; cover and refrigerate until ready to use.

Immediately before serving, top the dip with poppy seeds, sesame seeds, or dehydrated onions, if desired.

Storage note: This dip can be kept in a covered airtight container in the refrigerator for up to three weeks.

KEFIR FRUIT DIP

This dip is great to serve with a large platter of mixed fruit, such as strawberries, blueberries, canta-loupe, raspberries, and orange slices. It makes for a beautiful palette of colors—and it's healthy, too!

Makes 4 servings

1 cup Kefir Cheese (page 17)
½ cup chopped fresh pineapple
2 to 3 teaspoons honey or Sucanat, or 2 packets stevia

....

Combine all the ingredients in a food processor and pulse until smooth.

Transfer to a serving dish and serve.

Storage note: This dip can be kept in a covered airtight container in the refrigerator for up to three weeks.

TUSCAN KEFIR COTTAGE CHEESE DIP

Here's a savory version of our flavored cottage cheese. This is great for dipping fresh vegetables or crackers.

Makes 3 serving

1 cup Jane's Kefir Cottage Cheese (page 58)

5 cherry tomatoes, chopped

1 small green onion, chopped

2 fresh basil leaves, thinly sliced

1 teaspoon aged balsamic vinegar for serving

Mix together the cheese, tomatoes, green onion, and basil in a small bowl.

Transfer the dip to serving bowl and drizzle the balsamic vinegar over the top before serving.

Storage note: This dip can be kept in a covered airtight container in the refrigerator for up to three weeks.

CULTURED BORDER SALSA

The first time I made this salsa I completed the task, quickly cleaned the kitchen, and jumped into the shower. I didn't realize that the pepper-seed juice on my hands couldn't be washed off with soap and water. Needless to say, I started to feel the burn in places that are best described as delicate. When I finally realized I was going to need something milk-based to soothe the burning, I jumped out of the shower, grabbed a towel, and ran to the kitchen—dripping wet and praying that nobody would walk in. I poured plain kefir into a bowl while clinging to my towel, and then sneaked back into the shower to douse the affected areas with kefir. When I finally admitted to my husband what I had done, he said, "Now that's something I would have paid to see!"

The moral of my story? Wear your gloves when seeding a chile or pepper, or you may just light up your life in ways you never expected. Even with gloves, be careful not to touch your face, especially anywhere near your eyes.

Makes 1 quart; 32 servings

¼ packet Caldwell's Starter Culture plus 1 teaspoon sugar or fruit or vegetable juice, or 3 tablespoons Kefir Whey (page 17)

2 large tomatoes, coarsely chopped

½ large Vidalia onion, coarsely chopped

⅓ cup coarsely chopped cilantro

1 serrano chile, seeded and coarsely chopped

2 garlic cloves, minced

2 teaspoons cumin

¼ teaspoon Celtic Sea Salt, or to taste

⅛ teaspoon cayenne, or to taste

....

If using the starter culture, place ½ cup of water in a glass measuring cup and add the sugar or juice. Add the culture and stir until dissolved; set aside. If using kefir whey, add it when the recipe calls for culture.

Place the tomatoes, onion, cilantro, serrano chile, garlic, cumin, salt, and cayenne in a blender, and mix until smooth.

Add the culture to the tomato mixture, and place the salsa in glass jars and seal. Let the salsa sit on the kitchen counter for 2 days; then transfer it to the refrigerator.

APPETIZERS

Like dips, appetizers are a great way to introduce cultured foods into your diet. Appetizers aren't as scary as eating cultured veggies, because they come in small doses, and they can be part of a spread that also includes noncultured foods. Try a few of these recipes at your next party, potluck, or get-together.

PROBIOTIC PICKLE POPPERS

When she was ten years old, my daughter Holli asked, "Mom, why do you think you had me so much later than Maci and DJ?" She was referring to her 26-year-old sister and 24-year-old brother, and before I could answer, she said, "I think I know. You wanted to learn things, and you learned a lot by having me. And you know what else, Mom? I think when you had me I needed you. So we just needed each other. Don't you think?" I shook my head and grabbed her little hand and told her, "I really needed you, Holli, more than you'll ever know." Then she asked if she could help me cook something fun. She had a new apron and wanted to wear it because it had big pockets. That's the day this recipe was born.

A note before you begin: I recommend using Donna's Dills (page 196) in this recipe, but if you don't have them on hand, Bubbies Pure Kosher Dills are a national brand of naturally cultured pickles that can be used instead.

Makes 5 servings

5 tablespoons cream cheese

5 tablespoons Kefir Cheese (page 17)

5 slices pasture-raised ham

5 spears Donna's Dills (page 196)

Mix together the cream cheese and kefir cheese in a small bowl until combined.

Spread 1 heaping tablespoon of the cheese mixture evenly onto each slice of ham.

Roll each slice of ham around a pickle spear, and then slice into bite-size pieces.

KEFIR CHEESE BALLS AND TOMATOES THAT POP

This appetizer is a great variation of the classic caprese salad, but instead of fresh tomatoes and mozzarella, I use kefir cheese and cultured tomatoes. The cheese balls in this recipe are also delicious on their own. I keep a jar of them on hand pretty much all the time. Preserved in olive oil with green onion, the tomatoes take on a wonderful flavor that I love.

Makes 6 servings

1 cup Kefir Cheese (page 17)

1 stalk green onion, chopped

1 cup extra-virgin olive oil

18 Fermented Cherry Tomatoes That Pop (page 116)

1 tablespoon aged balsamic vinegar

6 to 7 fresh basil leaves, torn

Mix together the kefir cheese and green onion in a small bowl.

With either a medium cookie scoop or your clean hands, form the cheese mixture into 10 balls.

Place the cheese balls into a clean glass jar and cover with the olive oil. Allow them to marinate for at least 24 hours.

After marinating, place the cheese balls and tomatoes in a serving bowl, drizzle with a little of the olive oil from the cheese balls and the balsamic vinegar, and top with basil.

Storage note: The cheese balls in this recipe can be stored in a covered airtight container in the refrigerator for up to three months.

FRUIT AND CHEESE KABOBS

These colorful treats are great for setting a festive atmosphere. I made these for my daughter's birthday party, standing them upright in cups. They added an interesting vertical dimension to my cultured food presentation. And everyone loved them!

Makes 10 servings

20 Fermented Cocktail Grapes (page 119)

20 1-inch cubes fresh pineapple

20 fresh strawberries

20 1-inch cubes Colby-Jack cheese

On ten short wooden skewers, alternately thread grapes, pineapple, strawberries, and cheese, using two pieces of each ingredient. Serve.

FERMENTED OLIVE TAPENADE CROSTINI

A few years ago I visited my in-laws in Arizona and became enchanted by the most beautiful olive tree in their backyard. It looked like it was straight out of ancient times. I would sit and stare out the window at it and watch as the olives dropped to the ground. After five days of contemplating the tree, I came up with this recipe. I wrote it down and forgot about it—until I needed new recipes for this book. The recipe uses fermented garlic and olives, which are also a fermented food. They are cured in a brine to make them edible. If you love olives, you'll love this dish.

Makes 24 servings

1 cup cauliflower florets

2 medium carrots, chopped

½ red bell pepper, seeded and sliced

1 celery stalk, chopped

3 cloves Fermented Garlic (page 201)

1 teaspoon Celtic Sea Salt

1 teaspoon turmeric

1 teaspoon mustard seeds

1 teaspoon dill seeds

¼ teaspoon Caldwell Starter Culture or ¼ cup of Kefir Whey (page 17)

1 cup pitted black or green olives

¼ cup yellow banana peppers, packed in vinegar

2 tablespoons extra-virgin olive oil, plus extra for crostini

6 (¼-inch-thick) slices Donna's Sourdough Bread (page 129), cut from the largest part of the loaf

....

Place the cauliflower, carrots, red bell pepper, celery, garlic, salt, turmeric, mustard seeds, and dill seeds in a 1-quart canning jar.

Add the starter culture and cover with filtered water, leaving an inch or two of headspace to let the vegetables bubble and expand as they ferment.

Seal the jar tightly and let it sit on your kitchen counter for 2 days.

Once the vegetables have fermented, strain them and reserve the liquid.

Add the olives, banana peppers, and 2 tablespoons olive oil, and pulse until the mixture resembles a coarse paste. (You can add some reserved liquid from the fermented veggies if it is too thick.)

Preheat the oven to 350°F.

Cut each slice of bread in quarters.

Place the bread on a baking sheet and brush lightly with olive oil.

Bake for approximately 10 minutes, or until the bread is golden brown.

Allow the crostini to cool; then spread each piece with approximately 2 tablespoons of the olive tapenade.

Storage note: The olive tapenade can be stored in a covered airtight container in the refrigerator for up to one month.

STUFFED OLIVES

Do you love olives? I do, and green olives are my favorite, but stuffed green olives—now that's something to talk about. My mom loves these stuffed olives so much that I give her a jar every Christmas. So why not try them yourself? They're easy to make and oh, so delicious. Now if I only had an olive tree!

A note before you begin: Fresh dill is my choice for this recipe, but I know a number of people who have used other herbs. Feel free to use your favorites. Some folks have told me that they've replaced the garlic with Fermented Jalapeños (page 202) or Fermented Cherry Tomatoes That Pop (page 116) with tasty results.

Makes 10 servings

¾ cup Kefir Cheese (page 17)

2 tablespoons snipped fresh dill weed

1 teaspoon freshly ground black pepper

50 large pitted unstuffed green olives

12 cloves Fermented Garlic, chopped (page 201)

Mix together the kefir cheese, dill, and pepper in a small bowl until combined.

Stuff each olive with a small amount of the cheese mixture, filling each olive about ⅔ full.

Add enough fermented garlic to the olive to fill it.

Storage note: These olives can be stored in a covered airtight container in the refrigerator for up to two weeks.

CUCUMBER HUMMUS CUPS

These hummus cups are fun to make, and they're a delicious cool snack that's perfect for summer! Drizzle them with a small amount of lemon-infused olive oil, and they'll be even more refreshing.

A note before you begin: These cups are one of my favorite treats, so I make them all the time. They're perfect for everyday eating, and I usually just follow the method below. When I want to fancy them up for a get-together, instead of scooping the hummus with a spoon I use a pastry bag fitted with a large star tip to pipe in the filling. Either way, they're delicious.

Makes 8 servings

4 medium cucumbers

1 cup Fermented Hummus (page 72)

Chopped chives for garnish

....

Cut off the ends of each cucumber; then cut the remaining piece into 8 thick same-size slices to create 32 rounds of cucumber.

To create the cucumber cups, use a teaspoon or melon baller to scoop out the seeds to form a well in each piece. Scoop only about halfway through the cucumber.

Spoon about ½ tablespoon of hummus into the well of each cup, mounding it slightly.

Set the cups on a tray or serving plate and sprinkle them with the chopped chives.

Serve immediately, or tightly wrap with plastic wrap and store in the refrigerator for no more than one day.

SOAKED SALTED ALMONDS

Nuts and seeds are difficult for many people to digest because nature has structured them in a way that prevents them from germinating until the perfect conditions are present. This means that the absorption of nutrients is greatly reduced for those of us eating them. But soaking nuts—just like soaking grains—can minimize or eliminate this problem. The nuts are not only altered to make digestion easier, but the nutrients and minerals become more biologically available, so the amounts of the "good stuff" your body can absorb skyrockets. These simple, delicious almonds are what I use to bribe my video guys. I always double this recipe—and the almonds are usually gone by the end of the shoot.

Makes 20 servings

1½ to 2 tablespoons Himalayan salt

3 cups raw almonds

....

Add 1 teaspoon of the salt to enough filtered water to cover the almonds. Soak the almonds for 12 hours.

Drain; then rinse the almonds in a colander under cold running water.

Place the almonds in a bowl and toss with the remaining salt.

Put the almonds in a dehydrator at 115°F for 12 to 24 hours, or until the nuts are crispy and dry. You can also dry the almonds in an oven set at its lowest temperature. It should only take a few hours.

Storage note: These almonds can be stored in jars with tightly fitting lids in your cupboard for up to one month.

CHAPTER EIGHT

Main Courses

One of the questions I'm often asked is how to take cultured foods from a supporting act to the star role of the meal. In this chapter, I've presented some of my favorite main-course dishes that incorporate cultured foods—many of these even use foods from more than one category in this book! Once you get experienced at preparing cultured foods every day, you will be turning out your own creations. Please send me your ideas and recipes; I would love hearing about them. They'll inspire me, too!

KEFIR AVOCADO SOUP

This hearty soup is great as a main course—the healthy fat in the avocado fills you up quickly, and the fact that the soup is chilled means that you'll be getting the full benefit of the cultured foods. Remember, heat kills wholesome bacteria, so only chilled soups keep probiotics alive. *Viva sopa fría!* Pair this with sourdough bread to create a delicious summer meal.

Makes 4 servings

1 large avocado, peeled, pitted, and cut into large pieces, plus 4 thin slices for garnish

1 cup hot chicken broth

1 tablespoon freshly squeezed lemon juice

1 teaspoon onion powder

1 teaspoon garlic powder

¾ teaspoon curry powder

½ teaspoon Celtic Sea Salt

½ teaspoon freshly ground black pepper

½ cup Basic Kefir (page 15)

Place the avocado, broth, lemon juice, onion powder, garlic powder, curry powder, salt, and pepper in a blender, and pulse until smooth.

Allow the mixture to cool until just warm, then add the kefir and blend on low speed until combined, about 10 seconds.

Pour the soup into four individual bowls. Cover with plastic wrap and cool in the refrigerator for approximately 20 minutes.

Before serving, garnish each serving with an avocado slice.

SALMON WITH KEFIR GARLIC SAUCE

The creamy kefir sauce in this dish, which is flavored with pine nuts, garlic, and mustard, has a distinct Middle Eastern flavor that pairs well with fish, chicken, or vegetables. When I first created it, my husband was skeptical, but soon he was telling me how much he loved the sauce. And I love it, too—for so many reasons. Not only is it delicious, but it also reminded me once again how thankful I am for my husband's skepticism—and my family's pickiness—because it inspires me to make my food even more delicious. It makes me a better cook, for sure!

Makes 3 servings

For the Kefir Garlic Sauce

1 cup Basic Kefir (page 15)

6 tablespoons pine nuts

2 cloves Fermented Garlic (page 201)

¾ teaspoon Dijon mustard

....

For the salmon

2 teaspoons olive oil

1 pound skinless salmon fillet

1 teaspoon Celtic Sea Salt

½ teaspoon freshly ground black pepper

....

For the Kefir Garlic Sauce

Place all the ingredients in a blender and process until smooth.

For the salmon

Heat a grill pan over medium-high heat or preheat a gas grill.

Drizzle the olive oil over the salmon and sprinkle with salt and pepper.

Grill the salmon until the flesh is cooked through and flakes easily with a fork, about 6 to 8 minutes

FERMENTED CHECCA AND ZUCCHINI

Someone once asked me if I was Italian because I was always trying to get them to eat! While it's true that I often offer food, I am not Italian—but I do love pasta. *Checca* is a pasta sauce made from fresh uncooked tomatoes, and it's typically served in Italy in the summer. I substituted zucchini for the pasta and added the fermented veggies, because I'm always looking for ways to make food healthier and to add cultured foods.

A note before you begin: You can use a julienne cutter, mandolin slicer, or a vegetable peeler to prep the zucchini.

Makes 4 servings

2 pounds zucchini (about 4 medium, 9 to 10 inches long), cut into thin strands

5 tablespoons extra-virgin olive oil

15 Fermented Cherry Tomatoes That Pop (page 116)

15 fresh cherry tomatoes

½ cup grated Parmesan cheese

3 cloves Fermented Garlic (page 201)

8 to 10 fresh basil leaves

Celtic Sea Salt to taste

Freshly ground black pepper to taste

4 ounces fresh mozzarella cheese, cut into ½-inch cubes

. . . .

Sauté the zucchini with 2 tablespoons of the olive oil in a large skillet over medium heat for about 4 minutes.

Combine the tomatoes, Parmesan, garlic, basil, salt, pepper, and remaining 3 tablespoons of olive oil in the work bowl of a food processor, and pulse until the tomatoes are coarsely chopped.

In a large bowl, toss the zucchini with the tomato mixture and the cubes of mozzarella. Serve immediately.

KEFIR AND BROCCOLI SPROUTED PIZZA

Moms are always looking for ways to sneak more healthy food into their children's diets. It's just what we do. So when I figured out the recipe for this kid-friendly pizza, which incorporates sprouted grains, kefir, and cultured veggies, I was thrilled. And since broccoli is my little girl's favorite veggie, there are never any complaints when this shows up for dinner.

A note before you begin: The probiotic benefits of cultured foods are lost if the foods are cooked. For this pizza, you bake the crust beforehand, and then top with the remaining raw ingredients to keep the beneficial bacteria alive.

Makes 6 servings

Cornmeal

Dough for 1 Sprouted Pizza Crust (page 137)

1 cup Kefir Ranch Dressing (page 189)

2 cups Fermented Broccoli (page 118)

1 cup shredded Cheddar cheese

. . . .

Preheat the oven to 500°F. Lightly sprinkle a pizza pan with the cornmeal.

Roll out the pizza dough on a lightly floured surface to create a 12-inch round.

Transfer the dough to the prepared pizza pan.

Bake the pizza for 10 to 15 minutes until crisp.

Let the crust cool slightly until just warm.

Spread the dressing over the top of the crust.

Top with the broccoli and sprinkle with the Cheddar cheese.

SPROUTED PIZZA WITH KEFIR GARLIC SAUCE AND SPINACH

The kefir garlic sauce on this pizza is used in two ways—for flavor and for its healthy probiotics. While the sauce spread on the crust before baking loses its healthy bacteria because of the heat, it has a wonderful taste. The sauce used as a dressing after the pizza is out of the oven gives you a healthy probiotic kick!

Makes 6 servings

Cornmeal

Dough for 1 Sprouted Pizza Crust (page 137)

Kefir Garlic Sauce (page 89)

1 large red potato, sliced paper thin

1 small red onion, sliced thin

1 cup cooked chicken, chopped into bite-size pieces

1½ cups shredded mozzarella

2 cups fresh spinach leaves

Preheat the oven to 425°F. Lightly sprinkle a pizza pan with cornmeal.

Roll the pizza dough out on a lightly floured surface to create a 12-inch round.

Transfer the dough to the prepared pizza pan.

Evenly spread ¾ cup of the garlic sauce on the dough with a spoon, making sure to extend the sauce to the edges.

Layer the crust with the potatoes, onion, chicken, and mozzarella cheese.

Bake for 12 to 15 minutes or until the crust is golden.

Remove the pizza from the oven, and evenly distribute the spinach leaves over the pizza.

Drizzle the remaining garlic sauce on top of the spinach. Serve immediately.

KEFIR PESTO SANDWICHES

These sandwiches are great on the go—I even make them on my boat! You can check out a video of me doing this at culturedfoodlife.com. I made this video because I wanted to show people that incorporating cultured foods into their lives can be fun and easy, even on vacation.

Makes 1 serving

1 Multiseed Sprouted Grain Bun (page 133)

2 tablespoons Kefir-Pistachio Pesto (page 187)

1 thick slice mozzarella cheese

2 to 3 Fermented Cherry Tomatoes That Pop (page 116), cut in half

Slice the bun in half and spread the kefir pesto on both halves.

Fill the bottom half with the cheese and tomatoes, and close.

TORTILLAS WITH CULTURE

Tortillas can be the base for all kinds of quick meals. For lunch, I often just grab a tortilla, stuff it with cultured vegetables, and wrap it up. The combination here—with cheese, veggies, and turkey—is one of my favorite ways to get my probiotics.

Makes 2 servings

⅓ cup Kefir Cheese (page 17)

1 garlic clove, minced

2 basil leaves, chopped, or 1 teaspoon dried basil

2 Sprouted Tortillas (page 138)

4 tablespoons Maci's Cultured Carrots (page 109), finely chopped

1 spear Donna's Dills (page 196), chopped

2 slices turkey, chopped

½ cup shredded Monterey Jack cheese

. . . .

Mix the kefir cheese, garlic, and basil in a small bowl.

Spread half the kefir cheese mixture on each tortilla.

Pile each tortilla with half the carrots, pickle, turkey, and Monterey Jack cheese.

Roll up the tortillas and enjoy.

CULTURED VEGGIE SANDWICH

This recipe was inspired by a sandwich I had while eating out for lunch. The restaurant sandwich didn't have fermented foods, but it did have similar ingredients. So I substituted the hummus, cheese, and bread of that sandwich with their cultured counterparts, and voilà! My efforts were worthwhile—after I created this, I had it for lunch three times that week. I hope you love it as much as I do.

Makes 1 serving

2 slices of Sprouted Tomato-Basil Bread (page 131)

2 tablespoons Fermented Hummus (page 72)

1 ball Kefir Cheese (page 79)

3 or 4 Fermented Cherry Tomatoes That Pop (page 116), cut in half

4 thin slices cucumber

2 thin slices red onion

2 lettuce leaves

. . . .

Spread one side of each bread slice with hummus.

Dot one slice of bread with the kefir cheese and top with the tomatoes, cucumber, onion, and lettuce.

Cover with the other slice of bread.

FRUITY, NUTTY KEFIR SANDWICH

Before you look at the ingredients and say, "No way, no how!" let me explain. I eat kefir cottage cheese and fruit almost every day. It's ridiculous how much of this I eat. One day I scooped an apple slice in nut butter, and then piled my kefir cottage cheese on top. The combo of nut butter and kefir cottage cheese was so good it inspired me to think of other ways to use it. Putting it on a sandwich made the fusion of flavors even better. Don't knock it till you try it. And when you do try this—and realize how good it is—drop me an e-mail and let me know. I'll be expecting your message.

Makes 1 serving

1 cup Jane's Kefir Cottage Cheese (page 58)

1 cup fresh blueberries and strawberries

2 teaspoons honey or 1 teaspoon stevia

2 tablespoons nut butter (cashew, almond, or peanut)

2 slices Sprouted Whole-Wheat Bread (page 128) or Donna's Sourdough Bread (page 129), toasted

6 Fermented Cocktail Grapes (page 119), halved

....

Mix together the cottage cheese, berries, and honey in a small bowl.

Spread the nut butter on both slices of toast.

Spread the cheese and fruit mixture on 1 slice of toast.

Top with cocktail grapes and cover with the other slice of toast. Serve immediately.

CULTURED BORDER SANDWICH

This is a fun sandwich. It has tons of flavors and is really filling, plus I love how pretty it looks on a plate. I like to serve this with extra guacamole and salsa on the side—just for a little extra healthy bacteria.

Makes 1 serving

2 tablespoons butter

2 slices Sprouted Tomato-Basil Bread (page 131)

2 thick slices Cheddar cheese

½ cup Probiotic Guacamole (page 70)

½ cup Cultured Border Salsa (page 77)

½ avocado, peeled, pitted, and thinly sliced

4 Fermented Jalapeños (page 202), sliced

4 Fermented Cherry Tomatoes That Pop (page 116), sliced

½ cup spring lettuce mix

Warm a skillet over medium heat.

Butter both slices of bread, and place them butter-side down on the heated skillet.

Top each slice with a piece of Cheddar cheese, and cook until the cheese is melted.

Remove the bread from the pan, and spread the guacamole evenly over the melted cheese on both pieces.

Top one piece of bread with the salsa, avocado, jalapeños, tomatoes, and lettuce.

Cover with the other slice of bread, and secure the sandwich with a toothpick.

CHAPTER NINE

Side Dishes and Salads

Sides

Side dishes are the heart and soul of fermented foods. Many of these sides are used as ingredients in a number of dishes in this book, but they're also delicious on their own. The only negative I've found is that they can take up a lot of room in your refrigerator. If you're short on space, you can always move these cultured foods into smaller jars after fermentation to make room in your refrigerator. Once you get the hang of fermenting, you'll have many varieties and favorites that you will want again and again. Don't be mad at me if you wind up buying another refrigerator. I have four.

SAUERKRAUT

There is something special to know about sauerkraut. You don't actually need a culture to make it. The cabbage, when combined with salt, will make its own friendly bacteria when submerged in water. These good bacteria become dominant and crowd out any harmful ones. This is one of the easiest and most commonly made cultured veggies—perfect for a beginner!

Makes 3 quarts; 48 servings

1 large head of cabbage

2 tablespoons Celtic Sea Salt

Remove and discard the outer leaves and core of the cabbage.

Shred the cabbage to desired length, either by hand or using a food processor.

Pack the cabbage into a 1-gallon glass or ceramic container that can be securely sealed.

Cover the cabbage with filtered water, leaving 2 to 3 inches of headspace for the cabbage to bubble and expand as it ferments.

Add the salt.

Seal the container and let it sit on your kitchen counter, out of direct sunlight, for 6 days.

Check the cabbage every day to make sure it is fully submerged in the water. If it has risen above the water, simply push it down so it is fully covered. If any mold has formed because the cabbage rose above the water, do not worry. Remember, this isn't harmful. Just scoop out the moldy cabbage and push the rest back under the water.

After 6 days, transfer the sauerkraut to the refrigerator.

Storage note: The sauerkraut can be stored in a covered airtight container in the refrigerator for up to one year.

GOLDEN BEET SAUERKRAUT

This is one of the first recipes I made that my daughter Holli liked. Golden beets have a unique flavor. If you haven't tried them, you should. They are one of my favorite things to add to sauerkraut, because they give it a wonderful bright color and a slightly sweet-and-sour taste. I'm not sure what sunshine tastes like, but I'm pretty sure it's similar to this!

Makes 1 gallon; 64 servings

1 packet Caldwell's Starter Culture plus 2 teaspoons sugar or fruit or vegetable juice, or ½ cup Kefir Whey (page 17)

3 to 4 golden beets

1 large head cabbage

½ Granny Smith apple

1-inch piece fresh ginger

If using the starter culture, place 1 cup of water in a glass measuring cup and add the sugar or juice. Then add the culture and stir until dissolved. Let the mixture sit while you chop your vegetables—anywhere between 5 and 15 minutes. If using kefir whey, add it when the recipe calls for culture.

Peel and shred the beets, and add them to a 1-gallon glass or ceramic container that can be securely sealed.

Remove and discard the outer leaves and core of the cabbage; then shred the cabbage and add it to the container.

Peel and shred the apple and ginger, and add them to the container.

Add the culture and fill the container with filtered water, leaving 2 inches of headspace, as the vegetables will bubble and expand as they ferment.

Seal the container and let it sit on your kitchen counter, out of direct sunlight, for 6 days.

Check the vegetables every day to make sure they are fully submerged in the water. If they have risen above the water, simply push them down so they are fully covered. If any mold formed because the veggies rose above the water, do not worry. Remember, this isn't harmful. Just scoop out the moldy vegetables and push the rest back under the water.

After 6 days, place the sauerkraut in the refrigerator.

Storage note: This sauerkraut can be kept in a covered airtight container in the refrigerator for up to nine months.

APPLE SAUERKRAUT

I developed this recipe at Christmastime when I was looking for something pretty to add to my table. I took one of my favorite krauts and added a handful of dried cranberries for some festive color. It turned out to be not only beautiful but also incredibly tasty! You can also substitute other fruits, such as blackberries, grapes, or blueberries, but the cranberries are particularly pretty. With or without the added fruit, this kraut is delicious.

Makes 2 quarts; 32 servings

½ packet Caldwell's Starter Culture plus 1 teaspoon sugar or fruit or vegetable juice, or ¼ cup Kefir Whey (page 17)

1 small head cabbage

1 teaspoon Celtic Sea Salt

1 Golden Delicious apple

½ cup dried cranberries (optional)

Juice of 1 orange

....

If using the starter culture, place ½ cup of water in a glass measuring cup and add the sugar or juice. Then add the culture and stir until dissolved. Let the mixture sit while you prepare the other ingredients—anywhere between 5 and 15 minutes. If using kefir whey, add it when the recipe calls for culture.

Remove and discard the outer leaves and core of the cabbage; then shred the cabbage and place it in a large bowl.

Sprinkle the cabbage with the salt.

Shred or finely chop the apple, and add it to the bowl.

Add the cranberries, if using, to the bowl, and mix well.

Firmly pack the mixture into two 1-quart glass canning jars.

Add the culture and the orange juice.

Cover the mixture with filtered water, leaving 1 to 2 inches of headspace to let the cabbage bubble and expand as it ferments.

Seal the jars and let them sit on your kitchen counter, out of direct sunlight, for 6 days.

Check the mixture every day to make sure it is fully submerged in the water. If it has risen above the water, simply push it down so it is fully covered. If any mold formed because the mixture rose

DILLY PURPLE CABBAGE

Cultured foods are more than just healthy food. They're delicious, too. This vegetable mixture not only adds beneficial bacteria to the gut; it also puts a lot of color on the plate. And the garlic and lemon add zing to this recipe. I love adding a dollop of this cabbage to a salad.

Makes 1 gallon; 64 servings

1 packet Caldwell's Starter Culture plus 1 teaspoon sugar or fruit or vegetable juice, or ½ cup of Kefir Whey (page 17)

1 small head purple cabbage

3 carrots

1 small beet, any variety

3 garlic cloves

Juice of 3 lemons

3 tablespoons dill weed

....

If using the starter culture, place ½ cup of water in a glass measuring cup and add the sugar or juice. Then add the culture and stir until dissolved. Let the mixture sit while you chop your vegetables—anywhere between 5 and 15 minutes. If using kefir whey, add it when the recipe calls for culture.

Remove and discard the outer leaves and core of the cabbage. Shred the cabbage and place it in a large bowl.

Peel and shred the carrots and the beet, and add them to the bowl.

Add the garlic, lemon juice, and dill to the bowl, and mix until thoroughly combined.

Transfer the vegetables to a 1-gallon glass or ceramic container that can be securely sealed.

Add the culture and fill the container with filtered water, leaving at least 2 inches of headspace to let the vegetables bubble and expand as they ferment.

Seal the container and let it sit on your kitchen counter, out of direct sunlight, for 6 days.

Check the vegetables every day to make sure they are fully submerged in the water. If they have risen above the water, simply push them down so they are fully covered. If any mold formed because the veggies rose above the water, do not worry. Remember, this isn't harmful. Just scoop out the moldy vegetables and push the rest back under the water.

After 6 days, place the vegetables in the refrigerator.

LEMON-POPPY SEED VEGGIES

This is a family favorite at my house even though my youngest daughter, husband, and adult son are superpicky eaters. It's also really pretty. Because it is pureed, it can be used as a topping for a baked potato or even a sandwich as well as a side dish.

Makes 2 quarts; 32 servings

½ packet Caldwell's Starter Culture plus 1 teaspoon sugar or fruit or vegetable juice, or ¼ cup Kefir Whey (page 17)

½ medium head cabbage

1 large golden beet

4 garlic cloves

Juice of 3 small lemons

1½ teaspoons poppy seeds

1½ teaspoons dill weed

....

If using the starter culture, place ½ cup of water in a glass measuring cup and add the sugar or juice. Then add the culture and stir until dissolved. Let the mixture sit while you chop your vegetables—anywhere between 5 and 15 minutes. If using kefir whey, add it when the recipe calls for culture.

Remove and discard the outer leaves and core from the cabbage; then shred the cabbage.

Peel and shred the beet.

Place the vegetables in a blender or food processor; add the garlic, lemon juice, poppy seeds, and dill.

Add a splash of filtered water and pulse until smooth and uniform.

Pour the mixture into a 1-gallon glass or ceramic container that can be securely sealed.

Add the culture and then fill the container with filtered water, leaving at least 2 inches of headspace to let the vegetables bubble and expand as they ferment.

Seal the container and let it sit on your kitchen counter, out of direct sunlight, for 6 days.

Check the vegetables every day to make sure they are fully submerged in water. If they have risen above the water, simply push them down so they are fully covered. If any mold formed because the veggies rose above the water, do not worry. Remember, this isn't harmful. Just scoop out the moldy vegetables and push the rest back under the water.

SHELLEY'S CULTURED VEGGIES

A woman who came to one of my classes gave me this recipe. She has now become a dear friend, and she also did the beautiful graphics for my self-published book. These veggies are so delicious that I ate half a jar the first time I tried them! This is the cultured vegetable recipe I make the most; it's my husband's favorite.

Makes 1 gallon; 64 servings

1 packet Caldwell's Starter Culture plus 1 teaspoon sugar or fruit or vegetable juice, or ½ cup Kefir Whey (page 17)

1 large head green cabbage

6 carrots

½ white onion

½ Granny Smith apple

1 cup kale leaves or spinach leaves

2 tablespoons parsley flakes or chopped fresh parsley

2 tablespoons Bragg Organic Sea Kelp Delight Seasoning, or more to taste

2 teaspoons Celtic Sea Salt, or more to taste

1 garlic clove, minced, or more to taste

....

If using the starter culture, place ½ cup of water in a glass measuring cup and add the sugar or juice. Then add the culture and stir until dissolved. Let the mixture sit while you prepare the vegetables—anywhere between 5 and 15 minutes. If using kefir whey, add it when the recipe calls for culture.

Remove and discard the outer leaves and core from the cabbage.

Place the cabbage, carrots, onion, and apple in the work bowl of a food processor and pulse until grated. Transfer the mixture to a large bowl.

Chop the kale.

Add the kale, parsley, sea kelp seasoning, salt, and garlic to the large bowl, and mix the veggies until thoroughly combined.

Transfer a few handfuls of the mixture into a blender; then add 1 to 2 cups of filtered water and the culture. Pulse until a thick brine is created.

Pour the brine over the remaining veggies and mix thoroughly.

veggies. Make sure the veggies are packed tightly, leaving 2 inches of headspace to let the veggies bubble and expand as they ferment.

Seal the containers and let them sit on your kitchen counter, out of direct sunlight, for 6 to 7 days.

Check the vegetables every day to make sure they are fully submerged in the juice. If they have risen above the juice, simply push them down so they are fully covered. If any mold formed because the veggies rose above the juice, do not worry. Remember, this isn't harmful. Just scoop out the moldy vegetables and push the rest back under the juice.

The veggies will be a bit fizzy and sour when ready. Place them in the refrigerator.

Storage note: These veggies can be stored in covered airtight containers in the refrigerator for at least nine months.

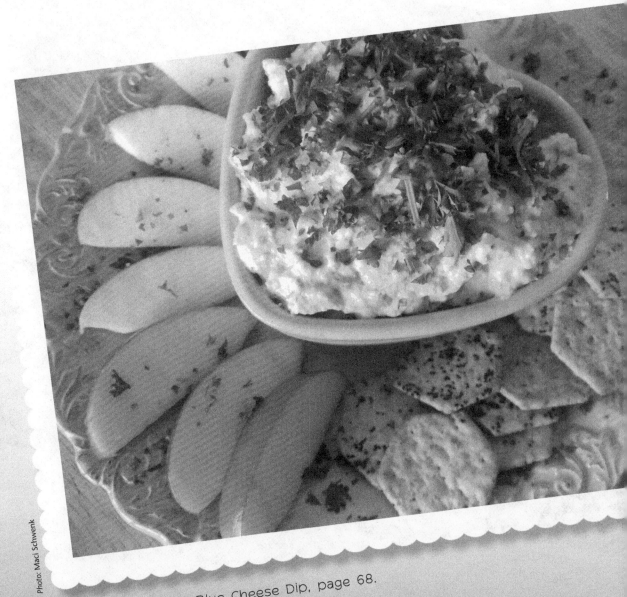

..., Kefir, and Blue Cheese Dip, page 68.

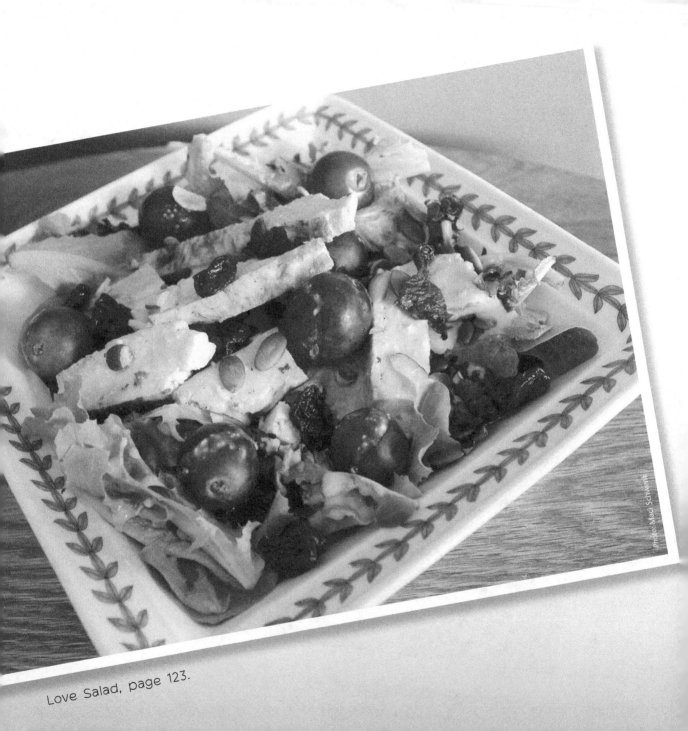

Love Salad, page 123.

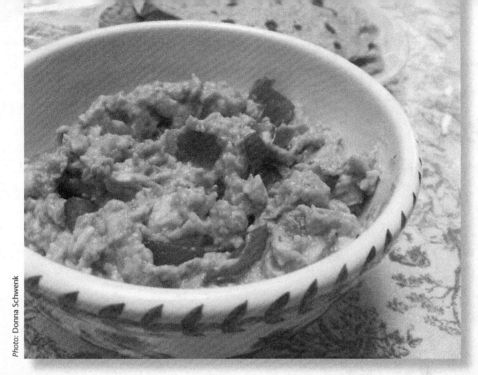

Probiotic Guacamole, page 70.

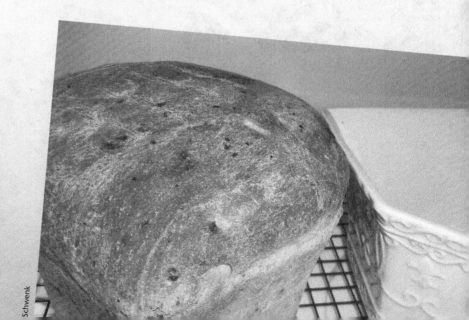

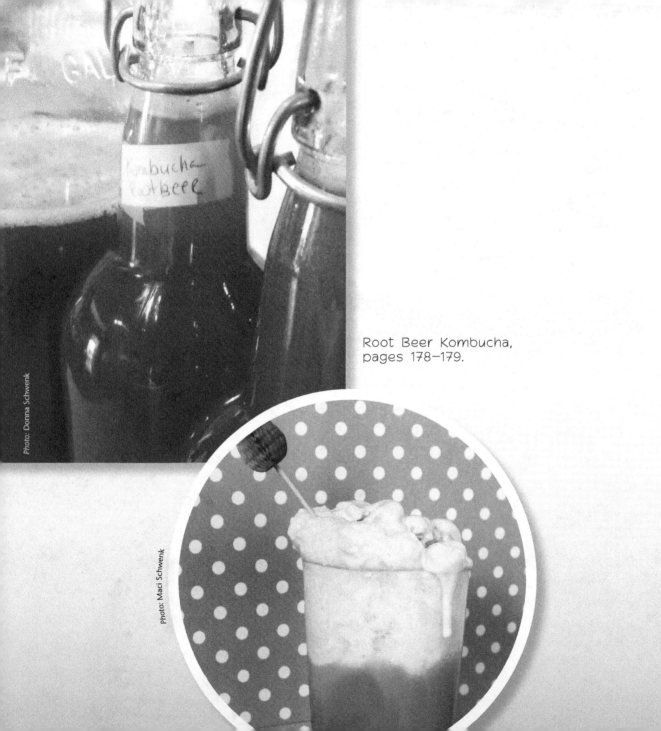

Photo: Donna Schwenk

Root Beer Kombucha,
pages 178–179.

photo: Maci Schwenk

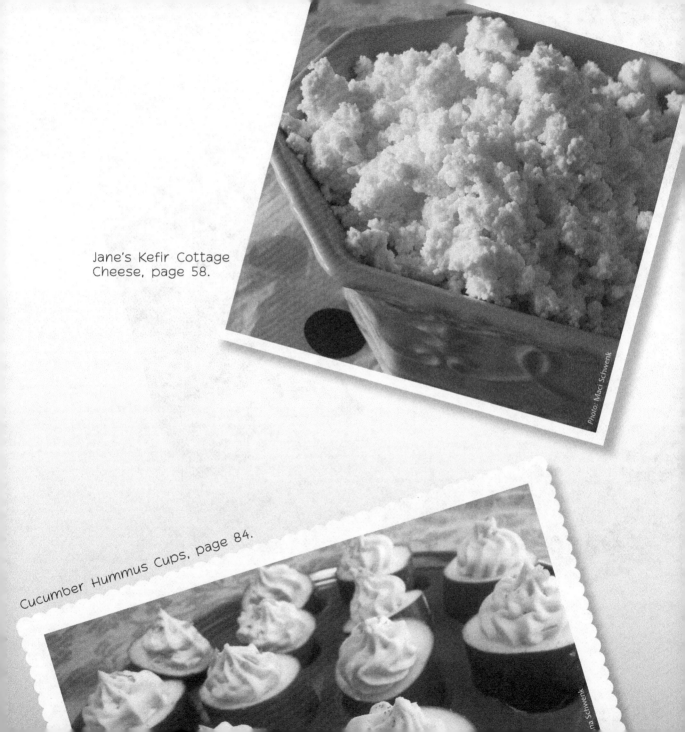

Jane's Kefir Cottage
Cheese, page 58.

Photo: Maci Schwenk

Cucumber Hummus Cups, page 84.

na Schwenk

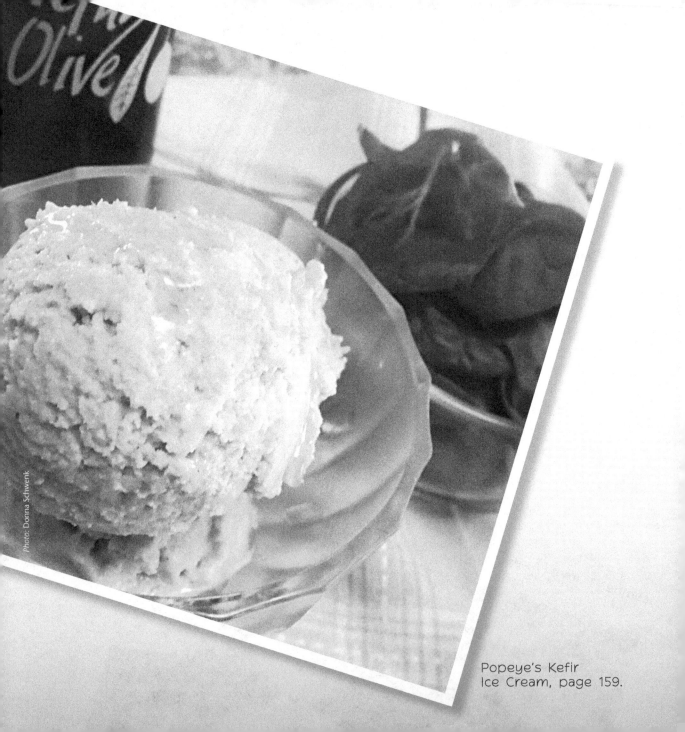

Photo: Donna Schwenk

Popeye's Kefir
Ice Cream, page 159.

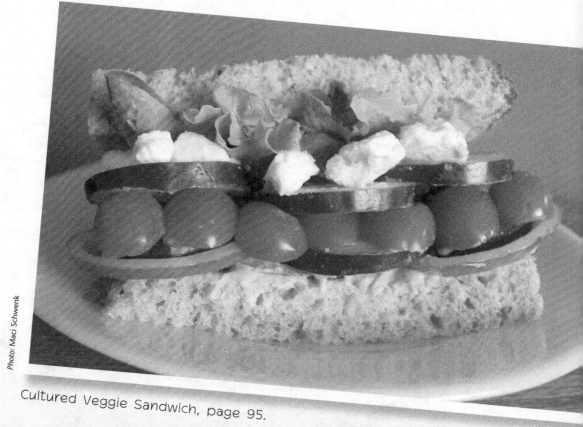

Cultured Veggie Sandwich, page 95.

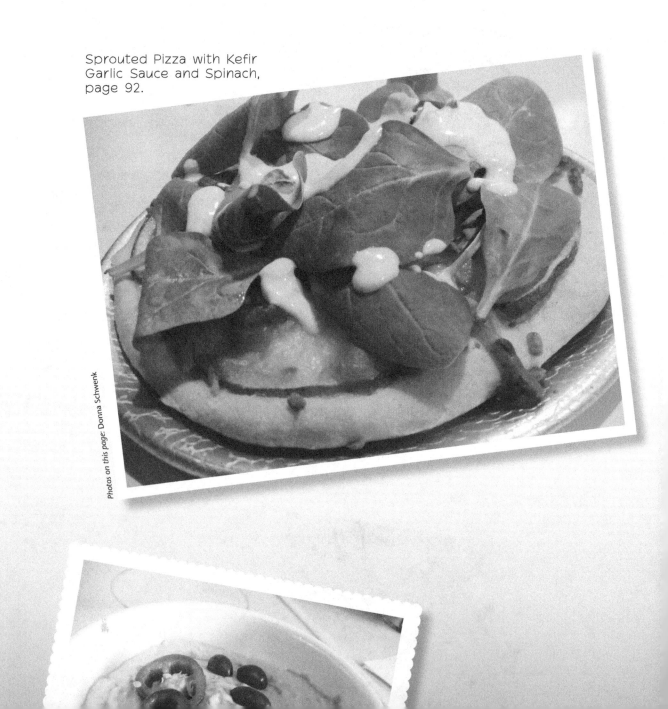

Sprouted Pizza with Kefir Garlic Sauce and Spinach, page 92.

photos on this page: Donna Schwenk

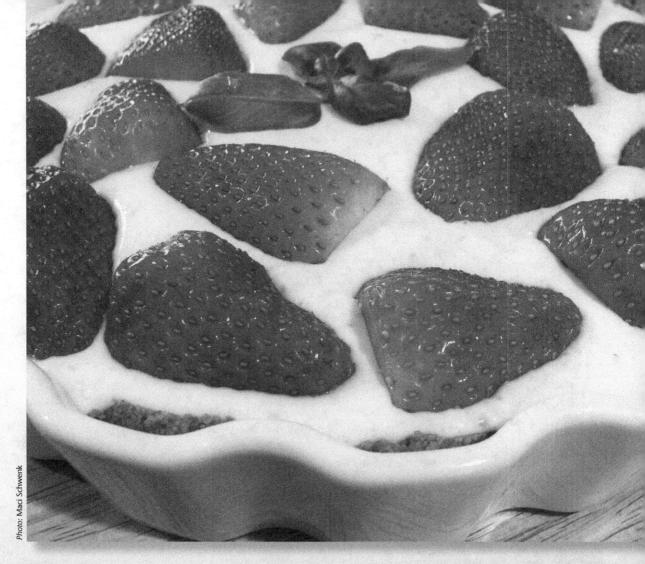

Strawberry, Lemon, and Basil Kefir Pie, pages 142–143.

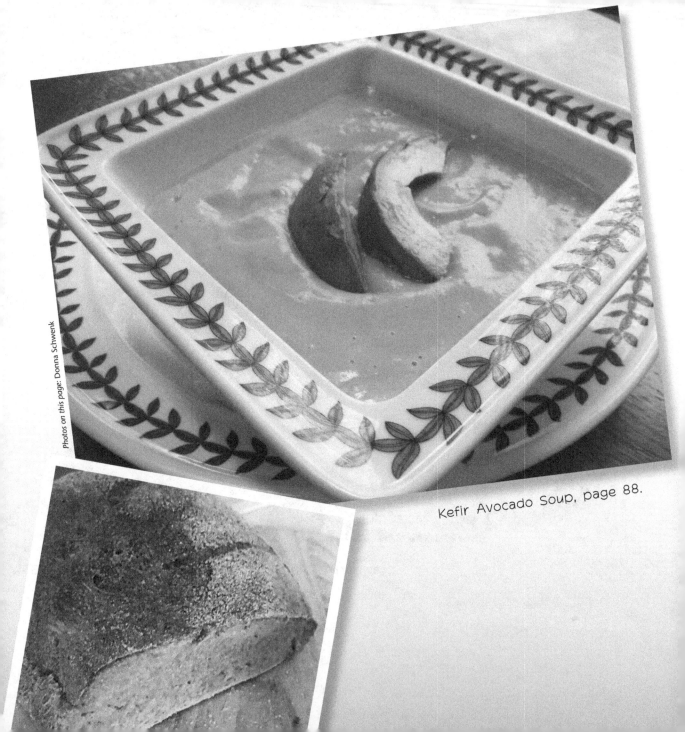

Kefir Avocado Soup, page 88.

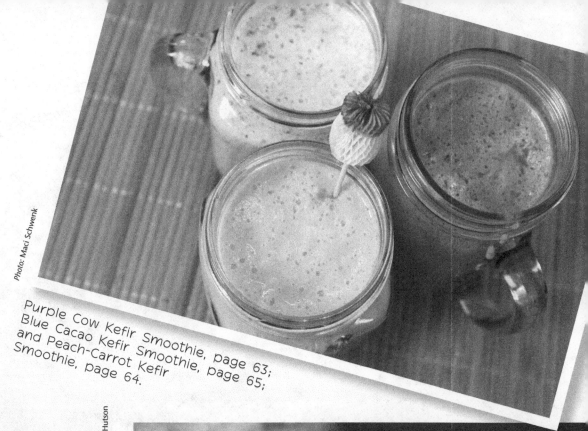

Purple Cow Kefir Smoothie, page 63;
Blue Cacao Kefir Smoothie, page 65;
and Peach-Carrot Kefir
Smoothie, page 64.

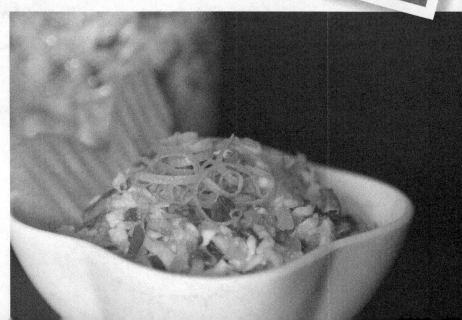

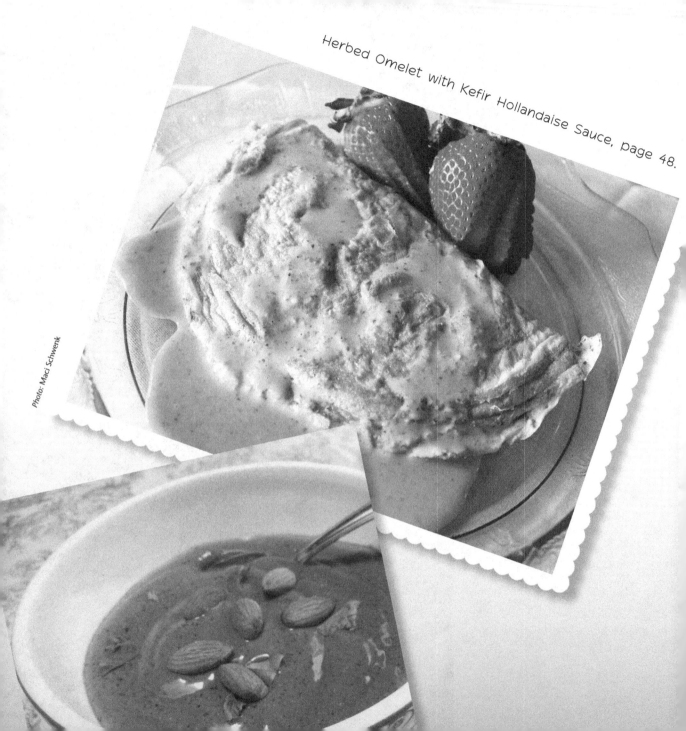

Herbed Omelet with Kefir Hollandaise Sauce, page 48.

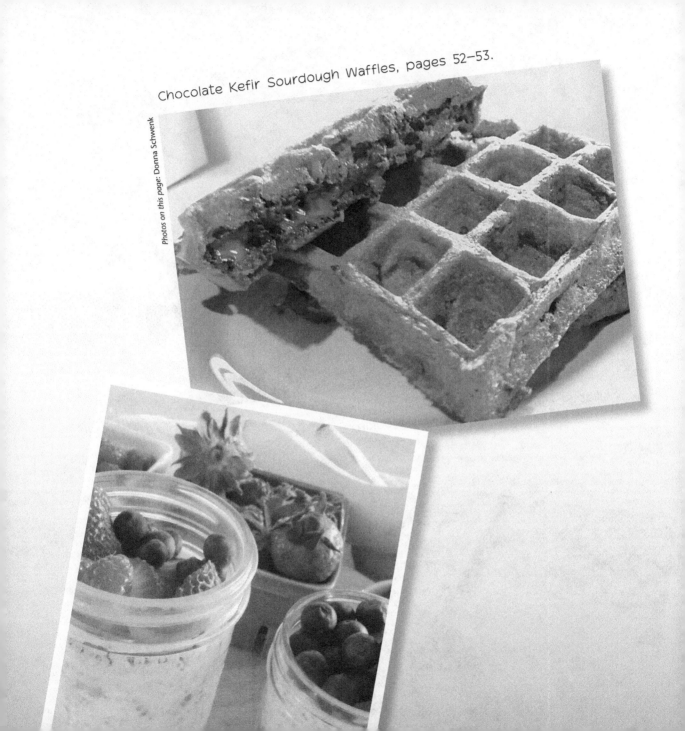

Chocolate Kefir Sourdough Waffles, pages 52–53.

Photos on this page: Donna Schwenk

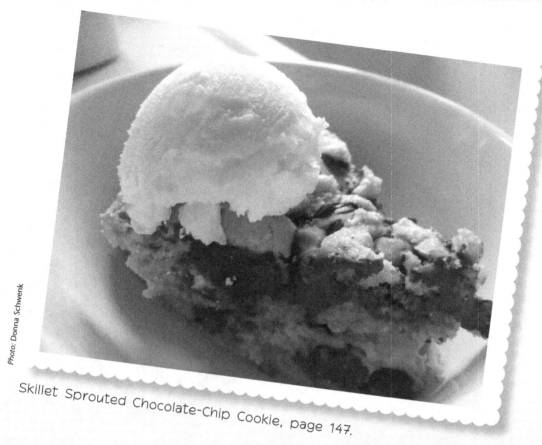

Skillet Sprouted Chocolate-Chip Cookie, page 147.

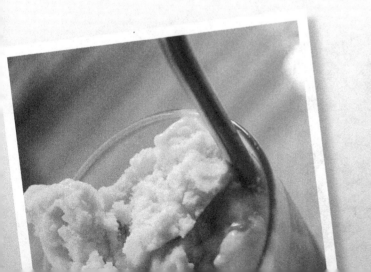

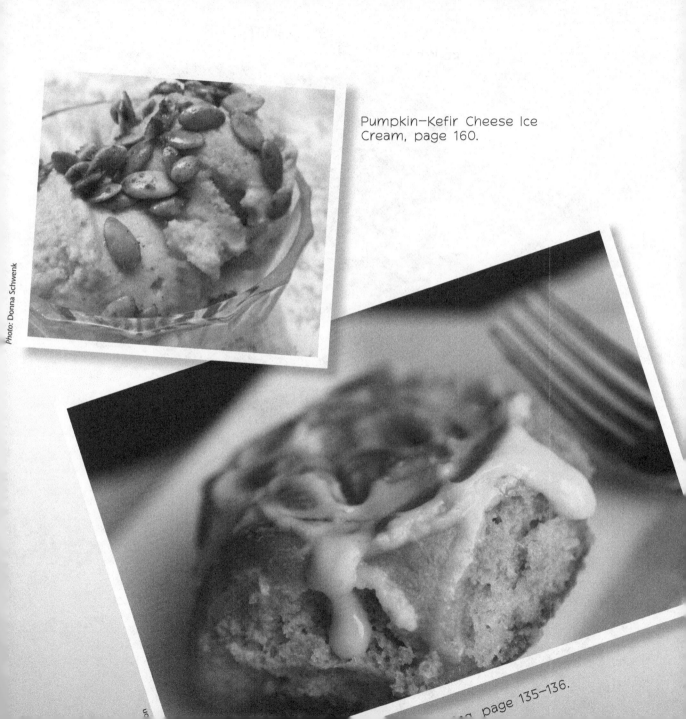

Pumpkin–Kefir Cheese Ice
Cream, page 160.

Photo: Donna Schwenk

page 135–136.

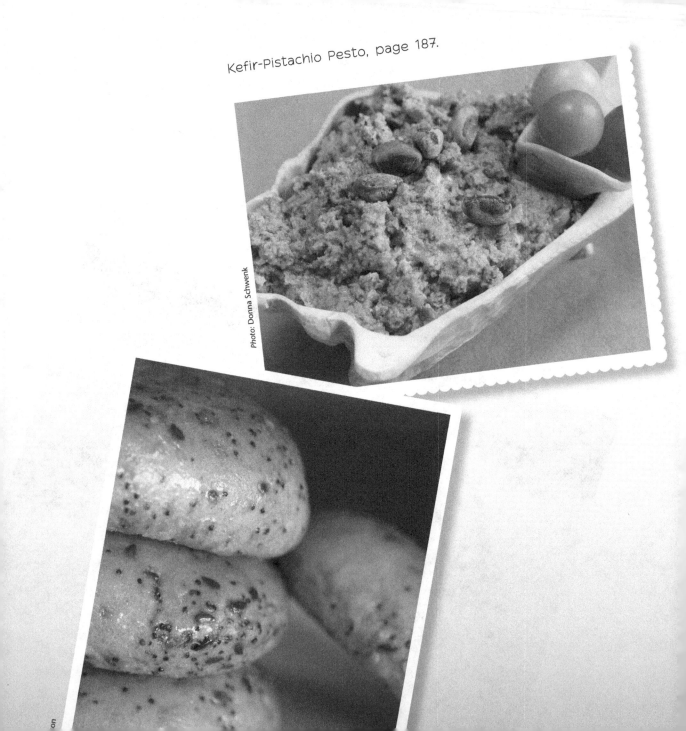

Kefir-Pistachio Pesto, page 187.

KIMCHI

Kimchi is an ancient food that Koreans have been perfecting for centuries. In fact, it is their national dish, and I'm sure that every family has its own recipe. My recipe is not as spicy as some, but you can adjust the seasonings to suit your taste.

Makes 2 quarts; 32 servings

½ packet Caldwell's Starter Culture plus 1 teaspoon sugar or fruit or vegetable juice, or ¼ cup Kefir Whey (page 17)

1 head Napa cabbage

1 bunch green onions

1 cup peeled and shredded carrots

½ cup peeled and shredded daikon radish

1 tablespoon peeled and grated ginger

3 garlic cloves

1 tablespoon Celtic Sea Salt

½ teaspoon dried chili flakes

....

If using the starter culture, place ½ cup of water in a glass measuring cup and add the sugar or juice. Then add the culture and stir until dissolved. Let the mixture sit while you prepare the vegetables— anywhere between 5 and 15 minutes. If using kefir whey, add it when the recipe calls for culture.

Remove and discard the outer leaves and core from the cabbage; then shred it. Place the cabbage in a large bowl.

Chop the green onions and add them to the bowl along with the carrots, radish, and ginger.

Peel and mince the garlic. Add it to the bowl along with the salt, chili flakes, and culture. Stir the ingredients until well mixed.

Transfer the vegetable mixture to two 1-quart glass or ceramic containers that can be securely sealed.

Press down firmly on the vegetables until all the juices come to the top; then cover the vegetables with filtered water, leaving at least 1 inch of headspace to let the vegetables bubble and expand as they ferment.

Seal the containers and let them sit on your kitchen counter, out of direct sunlight, for 3 days.

the veggies rose above the water, do not worry. Remember, this isn't harmful. Just scoop out the moldy vegetables and push the rest back under the water.

After 3 days, place the kimchi in the refrigerator.

Storage note: The kimchi can be stored in a covered airtight container in the refrigerator for up to nine months.

MACI'S CULTURED CARROTS

This is one of the first recipes my daughter Maci made herself. She is a great lover of cultured foods, and her enthusiasm for them is contagious. She ferments foods that I would never think of using, and she combines them in the most interesting ways. Maci even adds cultured veggies to her kefir smoothies! Second-generation fermenters are intense!

Makes 2 quarts; 32 servings

½ packet Caldwell's Starter Culture plus 1 teaspoon sugar or fruit or vegetable juice, or ¼ cup Kefir Whey (page 17)

8 large carrots

3 golden beets

1 large daikon radish

3 tablespoons chopped fresh basil or cilantro

....

If using the starter culture, place ½ cup of water in a glass measuring cup and add the sugar or juice. Then add the culture and stir until dissolved. Let the mixture sit while you chop your vegetables— anywhere between 5 and 15 minutes. If using kefir whey, add it when the recipe calls for culture.

Peel and shred the carrots, beets, and radish, and place in a 1-gallon glass or ceramic container that can be securely sealed.

Add the basil and the culture.

Fill the jar with filtered water, leaving 1½ inches of headspace to let the vegetables bubble and expand as they ferment.

Seal the container and let it sit on your kitchen counter, out of direct sunlight, for 6 days.

Check the vegetables every day to make sure they are fully submerged in the water. If they have risen above the water, simply push them down so they are fully covered. If any mold formed because the veggies rose above the water, do not worry. Remember, this isn't harmful. Just scoop out the moldy vegetables and push the rest back under the water.

After 6 days, place the container in refrigerator.

Storage note: These veggies can be stored in a covered airtight container in the refrigerator for up to nine months.

JICAMA WITH ORANGE

This is one of my favorite cultured dishes. Sweet, sour, and salty all at once, it has its own unique taste because of the orange zest and juice. This ferment is superbubbly and hisses in the jars in my refrigerator. I sold this at a store for a period and they couldn't keep it in stock and I couldn't keep up with the demand, so I decided to put the recipe in this book instead.

Makes 1 quart; 16 servings

¼ packet Caldwell's Starter Culture plus ½ teaspoon sugar or fruit or vegetable juice, or 2 tablespoons Kefir Whey (page 17)

2 small jicamas

Zest and juice of 1 small orange

2 teaspoons Celtic Sea Salt

. . . .

If using the starter culture, place ½ cup of water in a glass measuring cup and add the sugar or juice. Then add the culture and stir until dissolved. Let the mixture sit while you prepare the jicama—anywhere between 5 and 15 minutes. If using kefir whey, add it when the recipe calls for culture.

Peel and thinly slice the jicama.

Place the jicama, orange zest and juice, and salt in a 1-quart glass or ceramic container that can be securely sealed.

Add the culture and fill the container with filtered water, leaving 1½ inches of headspace to let the jicama bubble and expand as it ferments.

Seal the container and let it sit on your kitchen counter, out of direct sunlight, for 3 days.

Check the jicama every day to make sure it is fully submerged in the water. If it has risen above the water, simply push it down so it is fully covered. If any mold formed because the jicama rose above the water, do not worry. Remember, this isn't harmful. Just scoop out the moldy jicama and push the rest back under the water.

After 3 days, place the jicama in the refrigerator.

Storage note: The jicama can be stored in a covered airtight container in the refrigerator for up to nine months.

ROSEMARY FENNEL

This is delicious as a side dish, and is especially good served with fish. When you eat this dish, or any cultured vegetable, with a protein, it helps you digest the protein and absorb more nutrients than you would without it. The rosemary gives the fennel a clean, refreshing taste.

Makes 1 pint; 8 servings

⅛ packet Caldwell's Starter Culture plus ½ teaspoon sugar or fruit or vegetable juice, or 1 tablespoon Kefir Whey (page 17)

1 small fennel bulb

Zest and juice of ½ lemon

1 tablespoon fresh rosemary

1 teaspoon Celtic Sea Salt

1 garlic clove

If using the starter culture, place ¼ cup of water in a glass measuring cup and add the sugar or juice. Then add the culture and stir until dissolved. Let the mixture sit while you prepare the fennel— anywhere between 5 and 15 minutes. If using kefir whey, add it when the recipe calls for culture.

Thinly slice the fennel.

Place the fennel, lemon zest and juice, rosemary, salt, and garlic in a 1-pint glass or ceramic container that can be securely sealed.

Add the culture and fill the container with filtered water, leaving 2 inches of headspace for the fennel to bubble and expand as it ferments.

Seal the container and let it sit on your kitchen counter, out of direct sunlight, for 3 days.

Check the fennel every day to make sure it is fully submerged in the water. If it has risen above the water, simply push it down so it is fully covered. If any mold formed because the fennel rose above the water, do not worry. Remember, this isn't harmful. Just scoop out the moldy fennel and push the rest back under the water.

After 3 days, place the fennel in the refrigerator.

Storage note: The fennel can be stored in a covered airtight container in the refrigerator for up to nine months.

FLU PREVENTION CULTURED VEGETABLES

Here is a special recipe that I eat often during cold and flu season because of the extra vitamin C that it provides—the process of fermentation releases nutrients from the food, making them more bio-available for the body: for example, sauerkraut contains 20 times more bio-available vitamin C than fresh cabbage. I have seen cultured veggies knock out a cold or flu with a one-two punch, so this is the first thing I reach for when someone starts to feel sick. This is my flu prevention program. And remember, the juice is just as powerful as the vegetables. Just a spoonful of the juice can start you toward feeling good again, or, better yet, prevent you from getting sick in the first place.

Makes 2 quarts; 32 servings

½ packet Caldwell's Starter Culture plus 1 teaspoon sugar or juice, or ¼ cup Kefir Whey (page 17)

1 medium jicama, peeled

3 handfuls fresh spinach

½ small head cabbage, outer leaves and core removed

1 medium Granny Smith apple

1 small white onion

1 garlic clove

1½ teaspoons Celtic Sea Salt

Zest and juice of 1 large orange

If using the starter culture, place 1 cup of water in a glass measuring cup and add the sugar or juice. Then add the culture and stir until dissolved. Let the mixture sit while you prepare the vegetables— anywhere between 5 and 15 minutes. If using kefir whey, add it when the recipe calls for culture.

Shred or chop the jicama, spinach, cabbage, apple, onion, and garlic. Place them in a large bowl and sprinkle with the salt.

Firmly pack the vegetable mixture into two 1-quart glass or ceramic containers that can be securely sealed.

Add the orange zest and juice.

Add the culture and fill the container with filtered water, leaving 2 inches of headspace to let the vegetables bubble and expand as they ferment.

Seal the container and let it sit on your kitchen counter, out of direct sunlight, for 6 days.

veggies rose above the water, do not worry. Remember, this isn't harmful. Just scoop out the moldy vegetables and push the rest under the water.

After 6 days, place the veggies in the refrigerator.

Storage note: These veggies can be stored in a covered airtight container in the refrigerator for up to nine months.

RAINBOW CARROT STICKS

The first time I ate these, I was shocked at how something so simple could taste so good. The veggies are cut into bite-size sticks, and then fermented. They're a little sweet and a little sour—perfect for kids—but craved by adults, too. This works equally well with orange carrots, although it's not as pretty.

Makes 1 quart; 16 servings

¼ packet Caldwell's Starter Culture plus ½ teaspoon sugar or fruit or vegetable juice, or 2 tablespoons Kefir Whey (page 17)

6 or 7 rainbow carrots

Zest and juice of ½ lemon

....

If using the starter culture, place ½ cup of water in a glass measuring cup and add the sugar or juice. Then add the culture and stir until dissolved. Let the mixture sit while you prepare the carrots—anywhere between 5 and 15 minutes. If using kefir whey, add it when the recipe calls for culture.

Peel the carrots and cut them into matchsticks.

Place the carrots, lemon zest, and juice in a 1-quart glass or ceramic container that can be securely sealed.

Add the culture and fill the container with filtered water, leaving 2 inches of headspace to let the carrots bubble and expand as they ferment.

Seal the container and let it sit on your kitchen counter, out of direct sunlight, for 3 days.

Check the carrots every day to make sure they are fully submerged in the water. If they have risen above the water, simply push them down so they are fully covered. If any mold formed because the carrots rose above the water, do not worry. Remember, this isn't harmful. Just scoop out the moldy carrots and push the rest back under the water.

After 3 days, place the carrots in the refrigerator.

Storage note: The carrots can be stored in a covered airtight container in the refrigerator for up to nine months.

RAINBOW SWISS CHARD STALKS

This is a great way to use the chard stalks that might otherwise be thrown away. After the stalks have fermented, you can chop them up and add them to chicken or potato salad. The chard stalks taste a lot like celery, only milder in flavor, and these are much better for you because of all the healthy bacteria.

Makes 1 quart; 16 servings

¼ packet Caldwell's Starter Culture plus ½ teaspoon sugar or fruit or vegetable juice, or 2 tablespoons Kefir Whey (page 17)

1 large bunch of rainbow Swiss chard

1 teaspoon Celtic Sea Salt

½ teaspoon coriander seeds

If using the starter culture, place ¼ cup of water in a glass measuring cup and add the sugar or juice. Then add the culture and stir until dissolved. Let the mixture sit while you prepare the chard—anywhere between 5 and 15 minutes. If using kefir whey, add it when the recipe calls for culture.

Remove the leaves from the chard.

Add the chard stalks, salt, and coriander to a 1-quart glass or ceramic container that can be securely sealed.

Add the culture and fill the container with filtered water, leaving 2 inches of headspace to let the chard bubble and expand as it ferments.

Seal the container and let it sit on your kitchen counter, out of direct sunlight, for 3 days.

Check the chard every day to make sure it is fully submerged in the water. If it has risen above the water, simply push it down so it is fully covered. If any mold formed because the chard rose above the water, do not worry. Remember, this isn't harmful. Just scoop out the moldy chard and push the rest back under the water.

After 3 days, place the Swiss chard in the refrigerator.

Storage note: The Swiss chard can be stored in a covered airtight container in the refrigerator for up to nine months.

FERMENTED CHERRY TOMATOES THAT POP

These tomatoes are bubbly and fizzy and supergood. They may float around and bubble in the jar. Don't be surprised if they feel mildly carbonated when you bite into them.

Makes 1 quart; 12 servings

3 cups cherry tomatoes (enough to fill a 1-quart jar three-quarters full)

½ teaspoon Caldwell's Starter Culture or 3 tablespoons Kefir Whey (page 17)

....

Wash the tomatoes and place in a sterilized 1-quart jar that can be securely sealed.

Fill the jar with enough filtered water to cover the tomatoes, leaving at least 2 inches of headspace to let the tomatoes bubble and expand as they ferment.

Add the starter culture or kefir whey.

Seal the jar and let it sit on your kitchen counter, out of direct sunlight, for 4 days.

Check the tomatoes every day to make sure they are fully submerged in the water. If they have risen above the water, simply push them down so they are fully covered. If any mold formed because the tomatoes rose above the water, do not worry. Remember, this isn't harmful. Just scoop out the moldy tomatoes and push the rest back under the water.

After 4 days, place the tomatoes in the refrigerator and let ferment for 1 week more before serving.

Storage note: These tomatoes can be stored in a covered airtight container in the refrigerator for up to one year.

DILLY BEANS

These are great fun to make and are a zippy snack. I'll pull a couple from my jar to munch on when I'm hungry before dinner. These are not as sour as pickles; instead, they have a mild dill taste that kids love.

A note before you begin: This recipe calls for one garlic clove, but if you really enjoy garlic, feel free to add another clove.

Makes 1 quart; 16 servings

¼ packet Caldwell's Starter Culture plus ½ teaspoon sugar or fruit or vegetable juice, or 2 tablespoons Kefir Whey (page 17)

1 pound green beans

1 garlic clove

2 teaspoons dill weed

1 teaspoon black peppercorns

1 teaspoon Celtic Sea Salt

If using the starter culture, place ½ cup of water in a glass measuring cup and add the sugar or juice. Then add the culture and stir until dissolved. Let the mixture sit while you prepare the green beans—anywhere between 5 and 15 minutes. If using kefir whey, add it when the recipe calls for culture.

Wash, top, and tail the green beans and place them in a 1-quart canning jar or ceramic container that can be securely sealed.

Add the garlic, dill, peppercorns, and salt.

Add the culture and fill the container with filtered water, leaving 2 inches of headspace to let the green beans bubble and expand as they ferment.

Seal the container and let it sit on your kitchen counter, out of direct sunlight, for 3 days.

Check the green beans every day to make sure they are fully submerged in the water. If they have risen above the water, simply push them down so they are fully covered. If any mold formed because the green beans rose above the water, do not worry. Remember, this isn't harmful. Just scoop out the moldy green beans and push the rest back under the water.

After 3 days, place the green beans in the refrigerator.

FERMENTED BROCCOLI

When I first started culturing vegetables, I didn't think you could ferment broccoli. I'm not sure where I got that idea, but boy, was I wrong. Now this is one of my daughter Holli's favorite treats. Plus, it's a great addition to pizzas, pastas, and salads.

Makes 1 quart; 16 servings

¼ packet Caldwell's Starter Culture plus ½ teaspoon sugar or fruit or vegetable juice, or 2 tablespoons Kefir Whey (page 17)

3 cups broccoli florets

1½ teaspoons coriander seeds

1½ teaspoons juniper berries

1 teaspoon Celtic Sea Salt

If using the starter culture, place ¼ cup of water in a glass measuring cup and add the sugar or juice. Then add the culture and stir until dissolved. Let the mixture sit between 5 and 15 minutes. If using kefir whey, add it when the recipe calls for culture.

Place the broccoli in a 1-quart canning jar or ceramic container that can be securely sealed; then add the coriander seeds, juniper berries, and salt.

Add the culture and fill the container with filtered water, leaving 2 inches of headspace to let the broccoli bubble and expand as it ferments.

Seal the container and let it sit on your kitchen counter, out of direct sunlight, for 2 days.

Check the broccoli every day to make sure it is fully submerged in the water. If it has risen above the water, simply push it down so it is fully covered. If any mold formed because the broccoli rose above the water, do not worry. Remember, this isn't harmful. Just scoop out the moldy broccoli and push the rest back under the water.

After 2 days, place the broccoli in the refrigerator.

Storage note: The broccoli can be stored in a covered airtight container in the refrigerator for up to nine months.

FERMENTED COCKTAIL GRAPES

These grapes are unlike anything you have ever had. They are slightly spicy and taste great threaded on skewers along with cheese and veggies and other fruits. You've got to try them. They are superaddictive.

Makes 10 servings

2 cups seedless grapes

1- to 2-inch piece green onion, sliced

3 cloves

1 small cinnamon stick

¼-inch slice fresh ginger

1 garlic clove

½ teaspoon Celtic Sea Salt

¼ teaspoon Caldwell's Starter Culture or 2 tablespoons Kefir Whey (page 17)

....

Place the grapes, green onion, cloves, cinnamon stick, ginger, garlic, and salt in a 1-pint clean glass jar.

Fill the jar with filtered water, leaving at least 2 inches of headspace to let the grapes bubble and expand as they ferment.

Add the starter culture or kefir whey.

Seal the jar and let it sit on your kitchen counter for 3 days.

Check the grapes every day to make sure they are fully submerged in the water. If they have risen above the water, simply push them down so they are fully covered. If any mold formed because the grapes rose above the water, do not worry. Remember, this isn't harmful. Just scoop out the moldy grapes and push the rest back under the water.

After 3 days, transfer the grapes to the refrigerator.

Storage note: These grapes can be stored in a covered airtight container in the refrigerator for up to three months.

SALADS

We eat a ton of salad at our house. I try to have one almost every day. When you add a fermented dressing or a cultured veggie to the mix, your digestion is increased tenfold and you help your body absorb more of the vitamins and minerals. All fermented foods do this. It is why having fermented foods with your meal, no matter how small, is so important. It helps your body do things it was meant to do for you—and to do them with ease.

CKC (CULTURED KOMBUCHA COLESLAW)

This is a great coleslaw recipe, and no one will ever know that it's full of probiotics. I love taking this to a potluck or get-together—it's my way of spreading the benefits of healthy bacteria all over the greater Kansas City area.

Makes 6 servings

1 medium head cabbage, shredded

½ cup Maci's Cultured Carrots, drained of juice (page 109)

1 cup mayonnaise

½ cup Basic Kombucha (page 28)

½ cup honey

3 tablespoons Dijon mustard

2 tablespoons Basic Kefir (page 15)

1 teaspoon Celtic Sea Salt

½ teaspoon white pepper

....

Place the shredded cabbage and carrots in a large bowl.

Mix together the mayonnaise, kombucha, honey, mustard, kefir, salt, and white pepper in a small bowl to make the dressing.

Pour the dressing over the slaw and toss well to combine.

Storage note: This coleslaw can be stored in a covered airtight container in the refrigerator for up to two weeks.

BROCCOLI SALAD

Have you ever been to a potluck and had broccoli salad? I have had this many times and always loved it. And this version is so much better than any store-bought broccoli salad—it's a little sour yet a bit sweet with lots of crunch and good-for-you bacteria.

Makes 10 servings

3 cups Fermented Broccoli (page 118), drained, patted dry, and cut into bite-size pieces

1 cup cashews

½ cup Fermented Cocktail Grapes (page 119) or raisins

¼ cup chopped red onion

5 slices bacon, cooked and crumbled

1 cup Kombucha Mayonnaise (page 186)

1 tablespoon honey

....

Stir together the broccoli, cashews, grapes, onion, and bacon in a medium bowl.

Whisk together the mayonnaise and honey in a small bowl to make the dressing.

Pour the dressing over the broccoli salad and toss until well mixed.

Storage note: This salad can be stored in a covered airtight container in the refrigerator for up to two weeks.

CULTURED POTATO SALAD

I make gallons of this potato salad every summer. For a long time, my family didn't know it contained kombucha and kefir. In those early years of making cultured foods, the less information I gave them, the better! Eventually, the whole idea of eating cultured foods with every meal became the norm.

Makes 4 servings

1 pound red potatoes

¼ cup Kefir Cheese (page 17)

¼ cup Kombucha Mayonnaise (page 186)

1 to 2 tablespoons prepared horseradish

1 tablespoon chopped chives

1 celery stalk, chopped

Celtic Sea Salt to taste

Black pepper to taste

Cook the potatoes in a large pot of boiling water until fork-tender. Drain. When cool enough to handle, cut the potatoes into cubes. Place them in a large bowl.

Mix together the cheese, mayonnaise, horseradish, and chives in a small bowl to make the dressing.

Pour the dressing over the potatoes and mix until the potatoes are evenly coated.

Stir in the chopped celery, and season with salt and pepper.

Storage note: This salad can be stored in a covered airtight container in the refrigerator for up to two weeks.

LOVE SALAD

When I made this salad for a friend who was battling cancer, she said it was one of the best salads she had ever had. I told her it was the love I put into it more than the food itself. Love people, and cook them good food. That trumps all.

Makes 1 serving

2 handfuls spring lettuce mix

1 grilled chicken breast, sliced

½ cup Fermented Cocktail Grapes (page 119)

¼ cup feta cheese

1 tablespoon dried cranberries

1 tablespoon pumpkin seeds

1 tablespoon sliced almonds

¼ cup Goddess of Fermentation Dressing (page 191)

Place the lettuce, chicken, grapes, feta cheese, cranberries, pumpkin seeds, and almonds in a large bowl, and toss to combine.

Drizzle the dressing over the salad and serve.

PANZANELLA SALAD

This is my "I don't want summer to end" dish! I love going to the farmers' market on a Saturday to get fresh veggies to make this salad—and I love serving it, too. It is a colorful dish that's so gorgeous people often gasp when they see it. If you're like me, you'll save the sourdough bread cubes for last. They soak up the juices of the salad, and oh my, they are so delicious!

Makes 12 servings

6 cups cubed Donna's Sourdough Bread (page 129)

⅓ cup extra-virgin olive oil

¼ cup Basic Kombucha (page 28)

2 tablespoons juice from Fermented Cherry Tomatoes That Pop (page 116)

2 teaspoons minced garlic

1 teaspoon Celtic Sea Salt

½ teaspoon freshly ground black pepper

20 Fermented Cherry Tomatoes that Pop (page 116)

1 large seedless cucumber, quartered lengthwise and cut into 1-inch pieces

2 medium yellow bell peppers, seeded and cubed

1 medium red onion, halved and thinly sliced

⅓ cup chopped fresh parsley

. . . .

Preheat the oven to 400°F.

Arrange the bread cubes in a single layer on a baking sheet. Toast for 10 to 12 minutes until the cubes are evenly browned.

Meanwhile, place the oil, kombucha, fermented juice, garlic, salt, and black pepper in a large bowl and whisk together to make the dressing.

Add the tomatoes, cucumber, bell peppers, onion, and parsley to the dressing and toss to mix.

Just before serving, add the bread cubes and toss.

SPINACH SALAD WITH STRAWBERRIES AND KOMBUCHA-RASPBERRY DRESSING

This is a lovely salad to serve when strawberries are in season. It's not only delicious and healthy, it's elegant enough to serve for guests when you're trying to impress. Plus, it's easy. A win-win.

Makes 2 servings

3 packed cups baby spinach, washed and patted dry

½ cup fresh strawberries, hulled and chopped

½ cup pecans, chopped

2 to 3 ounces Gorgonzola cheese, crumbled

Kombucha-Raspberry Dressing (page 192) to taste

....

Divide the spinach between two plates, and top with the strawberries, pecans, and Gorgonzola. Drizzle the dressing over the salad and serve immediately.

CHAPTER TEN

Breads, Buns, and Other Doughs

They are many wonderful benefits to sourdough and sprouted breads. Both are made using techniques that were common until the mid-20th century. Prior to the 1950s, bread dough was fermented with a starter overnight, letting the bread have a long, slow, natural rise, so most bakeries ran two shifts of workers. Then corporations took over, and to increase profits, they introduced the fast loaf (three hours from start to finish), eliminating the need for a second shift of bakers. When bread is made the traditional way, the lactic-acid fermentation not only helps to preserve the bread, but also increases the nutrients available for our bodies. Today our guts are damaged due to processed foods, and we have trouble digesting gluten because of the way commercial bread is produced. You would be surprised what a difference sourdough or sprouted-grain bread can make. And there is nothing more satisfying than pulling a loaf of freshly baked bread from the oven.

SPROUTED WHOLE-WHEAT BREAD

I bake this sprouted whole-wheat bread all the time. It's full of flavor, great for sandwiches, and simple to make. I would recommend this for any beginner who might be just a tad nervous about baking bread. You won't be disappointed!

Makes 1 loaf

1½ cups warm water (105° to 110°F)

¼ cup olive oil

¼ cup honey

2¼ teaspoons dry yeast

2 teaspoons Celtic Sea Salt

4 to 5 cups Sprouted White-Wheat Flour (page 42)

Add all the ingredients to the bowl of a stand mixer fitted with a dough hook, and mix on low speed until the dough pulls away from the sides of the bowl and forms a ball.

Place the dough in a large greased bowl, cover with a clean kitchen towel, and let it rise until the dough doubles in size, about 1 to 1½ hours.

Punch down the dough, form it into a loaf, and place it in a greased loaf pan. Cover the pan with a clean kitchen towel, and let the dough rise until doubled in size, about 1 hour.

Preheat the oven to 375°F.

Bake the bread for 30 to 35 minutes, or until the crust is nicely browned.

Remove the loaf from the pan and transfer it to a wire rack to cool.

DONNA'S SOURDOUGH BREAD

This is the sourdough bread I make the most. It's slightly sour yet a tad sweet. The honey gives the starter something to eat, which makes the bread rise higher. If you're new to bread baking, I would recommend starting with this loaf, because it works so well. That being said, you will want to make it again and again, because it's just so delicious and easy.

Makes 1 loaf

9 ounces bubbly sourdough starter

1 cup warm water (105° to 110°F)

¼ cup olive oil

¼ cup honey

4 cups Sprouted White-Wheat Flour (page 42)

2 teaspoons Celtic Sea Salt

Cornmeal

Add the starter, water, olive oil, honey, and flour to the bowl of a stand mixer fitted with a dough hook. Mix on low speed until the ingredients are just combined. (You can also mix by hand.)

Let the dough rest for 10 minutes. Sprinkle in the salt. Mix on low speed for 3 minutes. (If mixing by hand, stir the dough with a wooden spoon for 3 minutes.)

Cover the dough in the bowl with a clean kitchen towel. Let it sit for 5 hours at room temperature (about 70°F).

After 5 hours, the dough should be doubled in size and moist and sticky. Stir the dough down with a couple of turns of your mixer or with your wooden spoon, and then roll it out on a lightly floured surface.

Fold the edges of the dough to the middle to roughly shape it into a ball. Dust the dough with flour, and using the fingertips of both hands, continue folding the outer edges of the dough to the middle until you have a ball. Don't use large amounts of flour to dust the dough, but keep enough flour on the dough to prevent it from sticking to your hands.

To make a round *boule* shape, place your hands on opposite sides of the dough, making sure you have some flour on the surface so your hands don't stick. Turn the boule in a counterclockwise direction, shaking it gently from side to side at the same time to encourage the dough to shape up from its flat state into a more tightly wound ball. Three or four turns should form a round ball. It doesn't have to be exact.

Let the boule rise for about 2½ hours, or until doubled in size.

Make sure your oven is preheated to 450°F when the dough is ready.

Slash the top of the dough two or three times with a sharp knife before placing it in the oven. Bake at 450°F for 5 minutes, then reduce the heat to 425°F. Bake the bread for another 25 minutes, turning the loaf halfway for even browning.

Remove the bread from the pan and transfer it to a wire rack to cool.

SPROUTED TOMATO-BASIL BREAD

This bread is so delicious—it's like a bowl of spaghetti in a single slice. It has the fresh flavors of basil and tomatoes, and it makes any sandwich taste simply divine. This bread also freezes well, so make extra loaves, if you wish.

Makes 1 loaf

2¼ teaspoons active dry yeast

1 cup warm water (105° to 110°F)

5 or 6 fresh basil leaves, chopped, or 2 tablespoons dried basil

¼ cup grated Parmesan cheese

¼ cup sun-dried tomatoes packed in olive oil, ground to a paste in a blender

1 tablespoon honey

1 tablespoon olive oil

1 teaspoon Celtic Sea Salt

2½ to 2¾ cups Sprouted White-Wheat Flour (page 42)

Dissolve the yeast in the warm water in a large mixing bowl. Stir in the basil, Parmesan, sun-dried-tomato paste, honey, olive oil, salt, and 2 cups of the flour. Stir in the remaining flour slowly—just until you have added enough to form a stiff dough.

Turn the dough onto a floured surface and knead until smooth and elastic, 3 to 5 minutes.

Place the dough in a large greased bowl, turning once to grease the top. Cover with a clean kitchen towel and let the dough rise in a warm place until doubled in size, about 1 hour.

Punch down the dough and knead on a floured surface for 1 minute. Place it in a greased loaf pan. Cover with a kitchen towel and let the dough rise until doubled in size, about 1 hour.

Preheat the oven to 375°F.

With a sharp knife, cut a large X in the top of the loaf.

Bake the bread for 35 to 40 minutes, or until golden brown.

Remove the bread from the pan and transfer it to a wire rack to cool.

Storage note: This bread freezes very well. To freeze, place the bread in a zip-close freezer bag, squeeze out any air, and seal the bag tightly. Store the bread for up to three months.

KAYLI'S CINNAMON SWIRL BREAD

I have never met a 13-year-old girl who has impressed me more than Kayli. I am proud to call her my friend as well as my aide in the making of this book. She has more wisdom than most women twice her age. The special way she designed this bread so that the cinnamon spirals in the middle is genius. Thanks, Kayli. I can't wait to see what you will do next.

Makes 1 loaf

Dough for Sprouted Whole-Wheat Bread (page 128)

4 to 5 tablespoons Sucanat or coconut sugar

3 tablespoons cinnamon

....

Add all the ingredients from page 128 to the bowl of a stand-up mixer fitted with a dough hook, and mix on low speed until the dough pulls away from the sides of the bowl and forms a ball.

After mixing, place the dough in a large greased bowl, cover with a clean kitchen towel, and let the dough rise until doubled in size, about 1 hour.

Place the dough on an oiled baking sheet, and shape it into a rectangle measuring about 20 inches by 6 inches. The dough should be about a ½-inch thick.

Mix the Sucanat and cinnamon in a cup. Sprinkle the mixture evenly over the dough.

Starting at one long end, tightly roll the dough toward the center, stopping at the middle. Then turn the pan around and roll the other long side until it touches the first rolled side.

Gently pinch the seam between the two rolled sides together and place the dough, seam-side down, in a greased loaf pan.

Cover the pan with a kitchen towel and let the dough rise until doubled in size, about 1 hour.

Preheat the oven to 375°F.

Bake the bread for 35 minutes, or until the crust is nicely browned.

Remove the bread from the pan and transfer it to cool completely on a wire rack before slicing.

MULTISEED SPROUTED GRAIN BUNS

I love my sister Danette. From the beginning, she said that every sign in the universe was telling me to pursue a career teaching people about cultured foods. She has always believed in me—and without her belief, you would not be holding this book in your hands. On one of Danette's visits, I made her a sandwich with one of these buns. She loved the bun so much that I send her some in the mail from time to time. Occasionally, the buns have sat in the post office until they were stale, but Danette never lets this bother her. She just makes them into an egg strata or a bread pudding.

Makes 12 buns

1 tablespoon sunflower seeds

1 tablespoon poppy seeds

1 tablespoon flaxseeds

1 tablespoon sesame seeds

1½ cups warm water (105° to 110°F)

2¼ teaspoons instant dry yeast

4 tablespoons maple syrup

4 tablespoons melted butter

1½ teaspoons Celtic Sea Salt

4 cups Sprouted White-Wheat Flour (page 42)

Put the sunflower seeds, poppy seeds, flaxseeds, and sesame seeds in a dry skillet, and stir them over medium heat. Let them toast, frequently stirring, until they start to pop. Don't let them burn. Remove the seeds from the pan and set them aside to cool.

Add the water, yeast, maple syrup, butter, salt, and flour to the bowl of a stand mixer fitted with a dough hook. Mix at low speed until a soft, wet dough forms; don't let it pull into a ball. (The softer the dough, the more tender the buns.)

Add the seeds and mix at low speed until the seeds are distributed throughout the dough.

Turn the dough into a greased bowl, cover with a clean kitchen towel, and let the dough rise until doubled in size, about 1 to 1½ hours.

Divide the dough into 12 same-size balls. Place the dough balls on an greased baking sheet. Cover with a kitchen towel and let the buns rise for at least 45 minutes, up to one hour.

Preheat the oven to 375°F.

NANCY'S HAMBURGER BUNS

This recipe is from my friend Nancy, who told me that I had to write this book. Although I was feeling very uncertain and hesitant, she convinced me that what I had learned needed to be shared. She is a light that shines the way for others to follow—plus, she makes some pretty amazing wheat buns. They're some of the best I've ever had.

Makes 12 buns

1½ cups warm water (105° to 110°F)

4 tablespoons maple syrup

4 tablespoons melted butter

2¼ teaspoons active dry yeast

1½ teaspoons Celtic Sea Salt

4 cups Sprouted White-Wheat Flour (page 42)

Add all the ingredients to the bowl of a stand mixer fitted with a dough hook, and mix on low speed until a ball forms that looks smooth. The dough should be soft and wet; do not let it form a hard ball. (The softer the dough, the more tender the buns.)

Transfer the dough to a greased bowl, cover with a clean kitchen towel, and let the dough rise until doubled in size, about 1 to 1½ hours.

Divide the dough into 12 same-size balls and place the balls on an oiled baking sheet. Cover and let the buns rise for at least 45 minutes, up to one hour.

Preheat the oven to 375°F.

Bake the buns for 15 minutes. For the best results, do not overbake.

Remove the buns from the baking sheet and transfer them to a wire rack to cool.

MRFENT'S CINNAMON ROLLS WITH KEFIR TOPPING

Chris, my web guy, known as MrFent on my website, has helped me with my business more than anybody this past year. He is responsible for making my website beautiful and for keeping me sane. When I think I can't do something, Chris tells me I can. And when I can't figure something out, he does it for me, and then shows me how to do it. Cooking is how I express love and appreciation to people, and since Chris loves my cinnamon rolls, I aim to have an endless supply.

Makes 12 to 15 rolls

For the kefir topping

½ cup Kefir Cheese (page 17)

½ cup mascarpone cheese

2 tablespoons honey

....

For the rolls

1½ cups warm water (105° to 110°F)

2¼ teaspoons active dry yeast

¼ cup olive oil

¼ cup honey

2 teaspoons Celtic Sea Salt

4 to 5 cups Sprouted White-Wheat Flour (page 42)

1 stick (8 tablespoons) butter, sliced thin

½ cup Sucanat or coconut sugar

1 heaping tablespoon cinnamon

Chopped walnuts or pecans, or raisins to taste (optional)

....

For the kefir topping

Mix all the ingredients together in a small bowl and set aside.

Put the yeast mixture, oil, honey, salt, and flour in the bowl of a stand mixer fitted with a dough hook, and mix on low speed until the dough pulls away from the bowl and forms a ball.

Transfer the dough to a large greased bowl, cover with a clean towel, and let the dough rise at room temperature (about 70°F) until doubled in size, about 1 hour.

Roll out the dough on a floured surface until the dough is a rectangle measuring about 15 inches by 9 inches.

Place the butter slices evenly over the dough.

Mix the Sucanat and cinnamon together in a cup and sprinkle the mixture over the buttered dough.

Sprinkle the dough with the nuts or raisins, if desired.

Starting with one long side, roll up the dough and pinch the seam together to seal.

With a sharp knife, cut the log into 12 to 15 slices.

Coat the bottom of a 9 x 15-inch baking dish with butter or oil. Lay the cinnamon rolls in the dish, cover with a kitchen towel, and let the rolls rise until doubled in size, about 45 minutes.

Preheat the oven to 375°F.

Bake the rolls for 20 to 25 minutes, or until nicely browned.

Remove the rolls from the oven and drizzle with the kefir topping while still warm.

SPROUTED PIZZA CRUST

You can vary the taste of your dough by using a basil- or garlic-flavored olive oil. For variety, I sometimes add a couple of tablespoons of Parmesan cheese to this dough. It's absolutely delicious.

A note before you begin: These instructions are only for the pizza dough. You get to be creative with whatever toppings you like. Just roll out the crust, layer with your favorite ingredients, and bake the pizza at 500°F for 10 to 15 minutes until the crust is browned and crisp.

Makes enough dough for 3 large (18-inch) pizzas

1¼ cups warm water (105° to 110°F)

2 packets active dry yeast

1 tablespoon honey

3 tablespoons olive oil

4 cups Sprouted White-Wheat Flour (page 42)

2 teaspoons Celtic Sea Salt

Combine the water, yeast, honey, and olive oil in the bowl of a stand mixer fitted with a dough hook.

When the yeast has dissolved, add 3 cups of the flour and the salt, and mix on medium-low speed. While mixing, add just enough flour, up to 1 more cup, to make a soft dough.

Continue to mix the dough until smooth, about 10 minutes, sprinkling it with flour as necessary to keep it from sticking to the bowl.

Transfer the dough to a large well-oiled bowl and turn the dough over to cover it lightly with oil.

Cover the bowl with a clean kitchen towel and let the dough rise at room temperature (68° to 70°F) for 30 minutes.

Divide the dough into three balls.

Use the dough immediately, or wrap it tightly in plastic wrap and refrigerate or freeze it for future use.

Storage note: This dough can be stored in the refrigerator for one week or in the freezer for two months.

SPROUTED TORTILLAS

These are supereasy to make and fun for kids who like to help in the kitchen. Make a bunch, because they get gobbled up pretty fast—and if they don't, they freeze well. One of my favorite ways to eat these is to spread a little butter on both sides of the tortillas and place them in a skillet over medium heat. While they are warming, I sprinkle them with cinnamon and Sucanat. What a delicious treat!

Makes 10 to 12 tortillas

2 cups Sprouted White-Wheat Flour (page 42)

½ teaspoon Celtic Sea Salt

3 tablespoons olive oil

⅔ cup warm water (105° to 110°F)

. . . .

Combine the flour and salt in the work bowl of a food processor. Add the oil and pulse to mix thoroughly. Slowly add the water through the feed tube while the food processor is running. Once combined, let the dough sit for 10 minutes, covered with a clean kitchen towel.

Turn the dough out onto a lightly floured surface, knead it a couple of times, and then pat it into a disk.

Divide the dough into 10 to 12 same-size pieces.

If you have a tortilla press (I highly recommend one; it's cheap and really handy), use it to flatten each ball before you cook it. If you're rolling by hand, use a floured rolling pin and a floured surface to roll each piece into a flat disk, 6 to 8 inches in diameter.

Heat a heavy ungreased griddle over medium-high heat.

Working with one at a time, toss the tortillas onto the griddle and cook each side until it begins to brown and puff in spots, about 1 minute per side.

Transfer the cooked tortillas to a plate and cover them with a clean kitchen towel to keep them soft and warm until ready to serve.

Storage note: These tortillas can be stored in the freezer tightly wrapped in plastic wrap for three months.

SPROUTED BANANA BREAD

I always have a loaf or two of this banana bread on hand. Banana bread is the best way to use over-ripe bananas. The bread freezes well, and it's perfect for an afternoon snack or as the base for the delicious Banana Bread French Toast on page 54.

Makes 1 loaf

2½ cups Sprouted White-Wheat Flour (page 42)

½ cup Sucanat

3½ teaspoons baking powder

1 teaspoon Celtic Sea Salt

1¼ cups mashed very ripe bananas (2 to 3 medium)

⅓ cup Basic Kefir (page 15)

3 tablespoons olive oil

1 large egg

1 cup chopped walnuts (optional)

Preheat the oven to 350°F.

Grease bottom of an 8 x 4½-inch loaf pan.

Mix together the flour, Sucanat, baking powder, and salt in a large bowl. Stir in the bananas, kefir, olive oil, and egg until well blended. Stir in the walnuts, if using.

Pour the batter into the prepared loaf pan and bake the bread until a toothpick inserted in the center comes out clean, 55 to 60 minutes for an 8-inch loaf, 5 minutes longer for a 9-inch one.

Remove the bread from the pan and transfer to a wire rack to cool completely before slicing.

CHAPTER ELEVEN

Desserts

The recipes in this section are some of my family's favorites. Parties, birthdays, and special events are the occasions for which these desserts were created. Ice cream is always a big hit at my house, so there are a few kefir ice-cream recipes that require an ice-cream maker. But there are lots of other sweet indulgences that need no special equipment to make. It's wonderful to be able to enjoy yummy homemade treats and know that they are good for you, too. It's important!

STRAWBERRY, LEMON, AND BASIL KEFIR PIE

The combination of strawberries with lemon and basil is like a taste of spring. The basil doesn't overpower; it simply imparts a fresh, sweet flavor. It's a lovely treat that complements the warming sunshine of the new season.

A note before you begin: I offer two crusts for this pie: Sprouted Graham Cracker or Gluten-Free. Both are prepared the same way, only the ingredients differ. In the gluten-free version, you can make the almond flour yourself by crushing almonds in a food processor.

Makes one 8-inch pie; 8 servings

For the sprouted graham cracker crust

1½ cups crushed Sprouted Graham Crackers (page 146)

4 tablespoons melted butter

For the gluten-free crust

1½ cups almond flour

3 tablespoons melted butter

3 or 4 chopped dates

For the filling

2 tablespoons unflavored gelatin

¾ cup milk

1 cup Kefir Cheese (page 17) or cream cheese

2 teaspoons Vanilla Extract (page 204)

5 to 6 basil leaves, chopped

Zest and juice of 1 lemon

1 cup Second-Fermented Citrus Kefir (lemon; page 16) or Basic Kefir (page 15)

4 tablespoons honey, Sucanat, or stevia

1 cup chopped fresh strawberries

For the crust

Combine all the ingredients in the work bowl of a food processor. Pulse 7 or 8 times until well blended.

Press the mixture onto the bottom and up the side of an 8-inch pie pan.

For the filling

Combine the gelatin and milk in a saucepan over medium heat, and cook until the gelatin has dissolved and the mixture comes to a boil. Set aside to cool for 5 minutes.

Once the milk mixture is cool, put it and the kefir cheese in the work bowl of a food processor along with the vanilla, basil, and lemon zest and juice. Process until combined, about 30 seconds.

Add the lemon kefir and sweetener to the cheese mixture, and process until combined, 15 to 20 seconds.

Taste the filling and adjust the sweetness to your taste.

Pour the filling into the crust and chill in the refrigerator for 1 hour, or until the filling is firm.

Before serving, spoon the strawberries evenly over the top.

PEANUT BUTTER AND CHOCOLATE KEFIR PIE

Whenever I get an idea for a recipe, it comes in a wave—I imagine that this is what people feel like when they are inspired to write music. Ideas start spinning in my head and take form within minutes. That's just what happened with this recipe. In fact, I made the pie so quickly that I had to go back and retrace my steps in order to write down the recipe.

Makes one 9-inch pie; 8 servings

For the chocolate piecrust

1 cup crushed Sprouted Graham Crackers (page 146)

1 tablespoon cacao or cocoa powder

4 tablespoons melted butter

....

For the chocolate ganache

½ cup heavy cream

⅓ cup organic 65% cacao chocolate chips or dark chocolate chips

....

For the filling

1 cup Kefir Cheese (page 17)

1 cup peanut butter

1 teaspoon Vanilla Extract (page 204)

4 tablespoons honey or Sucanat, or 5 teaspoons stevia

1 cup Kefir Whipped Cream (page 183)

Chocolate chips for garnish

....

For the chocolate piecrust

Place the graham crackers and cacao powder in the work bowl of a food processor and pulse until combined.

For the chocolate ganache

Pour the cream in a small saucepan over medium heat and cook until bubbles form around the edge of the pan.

Remove the pan from the heat, add the chocolate chips, and stir until the chips are melted and the ganache is smooth.

Spread the ganache over the chocolate crust; refrigerate the crust while you make the filling.

For the filling

Place the kefir cheese, peanut butter, vanilla, and sweetener in a blender and process on high until smooth.

Transfer the mixture to a bowl; then fold in the whipped cream, being careful not to deflate the filling.

Spread the filling evenly over the ganache.

Cover the pie with plastic wrap and place in the refrigerator for at least 3 to 4 hours, or until set.

Garnish with extra chocolate chips.

SPROUTED GRAHAM CRACKERS

These are delicious on their own, or you can use them to make graham-cracker piecrusts (Strawberry, Lemon, and Basil Kefir Pie, page 142; and Peanut Butter and Chocolate Kefir Pie, page 144). For a simple treat, spread the crackers with the frosting from the Brownie Cupcakes with Kefir Frosting (page 152).

A note before you begin: If you're baking the crackers to make into a crust, aim for the longer baking time. The longer the baking time, the crisper the crackers will be. Just make sure not to burn them!

Makes 12 servings

2 cups Sprouted White-Wheat Flour (page 42)

¼ teaspoons Celtic Sea Salt

¼ teaspoon baking soda

⅛ teaspoon baking powder

5 tablespoons melted butter

4 tablespoons honey

2 to 4 tablespoons water

. . . .

Preheat the oven to 350°F. Grease a large baking sheet or line it with parchment paper.

Mix together the flour, salt, baking soda, and baking powder in a large bowl.

Add the butter, honey, and just enough water to form a ball that is not sticky to touch.

Roll out the dough onto the prepared baking sheet.

Score the dough into 12 crackers with a sharp knife, then prick the dough all over with a fork.

Bake the crackers for 20 to 25 minutes.

Transfer the crackers, still in the pan, to a wire rack to cool completely.

Store the crackers in a sealed container in your cabinet.

SKILLET SPROUTED CHOCOLATE-CHIP COOKIE

For her birthday, my daughter Holli wanted a giant cookie, and this is what I came up with. It's so easy and so yummy that it just might become one of your go-to recipes. It's made in a skillet—no bowl to clean up—just stir and bake. It doesn't get any easier than that. There are lots of nutrients in this cookie and tons of deliciousness—especially when you top it with kefir ice cream. You'll be surprised by how filling it is.

Makes one 8-inch cookie; 8 to 10 servings

1 stick (½ cup) unsalted butter

1 cup Sucanat

1 teaspoon Vanilla Extract (page 204)

1 large egg

1½ cups Sprouted White-Wheat Flour (page 42)

½ teaspoon baking soda

¼ teaspoon Celtic Sea Salt

1 cup organic dark or semisweet chocolate chips

. . . .

Preheat the oven to 350°F.

Melt the butter in an 8-inch cast-iron skillet over medium-low heat.

Stir in the Sucanat and vanilla.

Remove the pan from the heat and let it stand until it is just warm, about 5 minutes.

Crack the egg onto the butter mixture, and use a fork to combine.

Add the flour, baking soda, and salt, and stir carefully until the mixture is smooth.

Add the chocolate chips and stir until evenly distributed throughout the dough.

Bake for 15 minutes, or until the cookie turns golden on top and around the edge, but remains soft in the center. Serve warm from the pan.

CHOCOLATE KEFIR ZUCCHINI CAKE

Making this cake with sprouted flour is ten times better than using store-bought flour. But using regular spelt flour is still better than going to the store and buying a cake. Store-bought cakes are filled with hydrogenated oils, preservatives, and chemicals. It is so much healthier—and tastier—to make it yourself, with or without sprouted flour. There are a ton of nutrients in this cake, not to mention all the love you put into it.

A note before you begin: The instructions for this recipe call for a 9 x 13-inch sheet-cake pan. If you would like to make a 10-inch Bundt cake, just increase the baking time by 10 minutes.

Makes 10 servings

For the cake

1 stick (½ cup) butter

½ cup coconut oil

2 cups grated zucchini

1 cup Basic Kefir (page 15)

1 cup maple syrup

2 large eggs

3 tablespoons cacao or cocoa powder

1 teaspoon Vanilla Extract (page 204)

2½ cups sprouted spelt flour

1 teaspoon baking powder

½ teaspoon Celtic Sea Salt

....

For the chocolate kefir topping

⅓ cup organic 65% cacao chocolate chips or dark chocolate chips

¼ cup Basic Kefir (page 15)

....

For the cake

Cream together the butter and coconut oil in the bowl of a stand mixer or in a large bowl with a hand mixer.

Add the zucchini, kefir, maple syrup, eggs, cacao, and vanilla, and mix well.

Combine the flour, baking powder, and salt in a separate bowl.

Add the dry ingredients, one cup at a time, to the wet ingredients, mixing until well combined.

Pour the batter into the prepared pan and bake for 40 to 45 minutes, or until a toothpick inserted into the center comes out clean.

Allow cake to sit for 10 minutes, then remove from pan and transfer to a wire rack to cool completely.

For the chocolate kefir topping

Place the chocolate chips in the top of a double boiler over low heat. Stir until melted.

Remove from the heat. When the chocolate is warm, but not hot (100°F or less), add the kefir and stir until well combined.

Drizzle the topping over the cool cake.

LEMON KEFIR YULE LOG

Around Christmastime, I bring this cake and my kefir eggnog to all of the cultured food classes I teach. They help the class get into the spirit of the season as the participants learn to make their own cultured veggies and kefir soda. While they enjoy the cake, I enjoy watching the information about cultured foods spread. For me, it's nearly as exciting as opening presents on Christmas morning.

Makes 12 servings

For the cake dough

6 large eggs, separated

⅓ cup Kefir Cheese (page 17)

Pinch of salt

For the filling

½ cup Kefir Cheese (page 17)

3 ounces cream cheese

1 avocado, pitted and peeled

Zest and juice of 1 lemon

4 tablespoons honey

½ cup chopped pistachio nuts

¼ cup dried cranberries

For the cake dough

Preheat the oven to 300°F. Cut a piece of parchment paper into an 11 x 15-inch rectangle and place it on a large rimmed baking sheet.

Whisk together the egg yolks, kefir cheese, and salt in a mixing bowl. Set aside.

Beat the egg whites in a separate bowl with an electric hand mixer on high speed until stiff peaks form when the beaters are lifted.

Remove the cake from the oven when lightly golden brown. Lift the parchment paper, with cake on it, and transfer to a wire rack to cool.

For the filling

While the cake is cooling, place the kefir cheese, cream cheese, avocado, lemon zest and juice, and honey in the work bowl of a food processor and pulse until well combined.

Spread the filling evenly over the cake and sprinkle with the pistachios and cranberries.

Starting at one short side, roll up the cake jelly-roll fashion; then wrap in plastic wrap.

Chill the cake in the refrigerator until ready to serve.

BROWNIE CUPCAKES WITH KEFIR FROSTING

These brownie cupcakes are gluten-free and supermoist. I've gotten more compliments on these than for any other cupcakes I've ever made—especially the frosting, which melts in your mouth. My good friend Nancy said she loved the frosting so much that she wanted to spread it all over her face. I'm not sure what that means, but I think it was a compliment. Probiotic frosting or face cream: your choice.

A note before you begin: This recipe calls for walnut or pecan meal. Many people aren't familiar with nut meals, but they are easy to make. Simply soak the nuts overnight and drain; then pulse them in a food processor until finely ground.

Makes 12 servings

For the cupcakes

1¾ cups walnut or pecan meal

¾ cup cocoa powder

1½ teaspoons baking powder

1½ teaspoons baking soda

½ teaspoon Celtic Sea Salt

2 large eggs

1 cup coconut milk

½ cup honey

2 teaspoons Vanilla Extract (page 204)

⅓ cup coconut oil, melted

....

For the kefir frosting

¾ cup coconut sugar or Sucanat

½ cup Kefir Cheese (page 17)

One 8-ounce block cream cheese, softened

1 ripe avocado

⅔ cup coconut cream or butter

For the cupcakes

Preheat the oven to 350°F. Line a 12-cup muffin pan with paper liners.

Mix together the walnut or pecan meal, cocoa powder, baking powder, baking soda, and salt in a large bowl. Set aside.

Whisk the eggs for 1 minute in another bowl. Add the coconut milk, honey, and vanilla, and whisk until combined.

Stir in the coconut oil and whisk until all the wet ingredients are combined.

Stir the wet ingredients into the dry, and mix well. Be sure to scrape the side and bottom of the bowl so that no dry ingredients remain. The batter will appear thinner than the usual cupcake batter.

Fill muffin cups halfway with batter.

Bake the cupcakes for 25 to 30 minutes, or until a toothpick inserted in the centers comes out clean.

Remove the cupcakes from the pan and transfer them to a wire rack to cool.

For the kefir frosting

While the cupcakes are baking, place the coconut sugar in a spice mill or blender, and grind to a powder. Set aside.

Place the kefir cheese, cream cheese, avocado, and coconut sugar in the work bowl of a food processor or into a large mixing bowl. If using a food processor, pulse until smooth. If using a hand mixer, beat until smooth, approximately 2 minutes.

Add the coconut cream, rum vanilla, and salt, and beat until smooth.

Spread the frosting evenly on the cool cupcakes.

CHOCOLATE KEFIR WHOOPIE PIES

When my little girl Holli turned ten, I made whoopie pies for her birthday party. Watching her guests walk around with these little pies was really cute. Hearing Holli explain that these treats were kefir pies was even cuter. The kids didn't care that the pies had kefir in them; they only cared that they tasted so good.

Makes 12 servings

2 cups Sprouted White-Wheat Flour (page 42)

½ cup Dutch-process cocoa powder

1¼ teaspoons baking soda

1 teaspoon Celtic Sea Salt

1 cup well shaken Basic Kefir (page 15)

1 teaspoon Vanilla Extract (page 204)

1 stick (½ cup) unsalted butter, softened

1 cup Sucanat or honey

1 large egg

Kefir Whipped Cream (page 183)

....

Preheat the oven to 350°F. Grease two large baking sheets. Set oven racks in upper and lower thirds of the oven.

Mix together the flour, cocoa, baking soda, and salt in a medium bowl until combined.

Stir together the kefir and vanilla in a small bowl.

Beat together the butter and Sucanat in the bowl of a stand mixer at medium-high speed until pale and fluffy, about 3 minutes. If using a hand mixer, beat for 5 minutes.

Add the egg and continue to beat at medium-high until well combined.

Reduce mixer speed to low and alternately mix in portions of the flour mixture and the kefir mixture until well blended, occasionally scraping down the side of the bowl.

Spoon ¼ cup of batter for each pie onto the prepared baking sheets, allowing about 2 inches between each pie, to make a total of 24 pies.

Bake the pies for 11 to 13 minutes, switching the positions of the baking sheets after 6 minutes, until the tops are puffed and spring back when touched.

KEFIR-COVERED STRAWBERRIES

This is the easiest recipe in the book. You can freeze the strawberries for an event, or just eat them one by one out of the freezer as I do. Yep, I did eat an entire pan one afternoon. I told myself I would only have one more until . . . there were no more!

A note before you begin: You can do all sorts of things with the coated berries: Roll them in nuts or shredded coconut before you freeze them, use flavored kefir for the coating, or simply create an extra-thick shell by freezing the berries for one hour, and then redipping them. Be creative!

Makes 12 strawberries

1 cup Basic Kefir (page 15)

2 tablespoons honey or Sucanat, or 2 teaspoons stevia

12 large strawberries, tops intact

Line a baking sheet with parchment or wax paper.

Mix together the kefir and the sweetener in a small bowl.

Dip the strawberries in the kefir, place them on the prepared baking sheet, and freeze them for at least 30 minutes.

KEFIR ICE CREAM WITH MAGICAL CHOCOLATE TOPPING

Have you ever had a chocolate-dipped ice-cream cone? Well, now you can have it again! And this time, it'll have some great health benefits! The topping in this recipe is made with coconut oil, which is a staple in our house. It has caprylic acid, a candida killer, so when my daughter was having problems with a yeast flare-up, she had coconut oil every day. Coconut oil helps the digestive tract absorb other nutrients, plus it raises metabolism and stimulates the thyroid. This is not just lip service; I've witnessed the results.

Makes 6 to 8 servings

For the ice cream

1½ cups milk

1½ cups Basic Kefir (page 15)

½ cup honey

3 egg yolks

1 teaspoon Vanilla Extract (page 204)

....

For the chocolate topping

¾ cup dark chocolate, cut into small pieces

½ cup coconut oil

....

For the ice cream

Place all the ingredients in a blender and process on high for about 1 minute, or until smooth.

Chill in the refrigerator for 20 minutes.

Pour the chilled mixture into your ice-cream maker and process according to the manufacturer's instructions.

For the chocolate topping

Combine the chocolate and coconut oil in a saucepan over low heat, and stir until the chocolate is almost, but not entirely, melted.

Drizzle the topping slowly over cold ice cream. The coconut oil will harden just after it hits the ice cream.

Storage note: Any extra chocolate topping can be poured into a squeeze bottle or glass jar and stored for up to three months. It does not need to be refrigerated. In the summer months, it will be a liquid at room temperature, and in the winter months, it will likely be solid. (Coconut oil becomes solid at 70°F.) If the topping hardens, place the container in a pan of warm water until it softens.

COCONUT KEFIR ICE CREAM WITH MANGO SOUP

When I went to the Caribbean, I thought I had died and gone to heaven. The water was the bluest blue I had ever seen. And the food was wonderful—coconut was in everything, and I love coconut. When I got home, I played Jimmy Buffett tunes and made coconut dishes for an entire year. It was during that period that I came up with this tropical dessert. Just like the Caribbean, it's heavenly.

Makes 1 pint; 2 servings

For the ice cream

1¾ cups coconut milk

½ cup Second-Fermented Citrus Kefir (orange; page 16) or Basic Kefir (page 15)

3 to 4 tablespoons honey or 3 to 4 teaspoons stevia

1 teaspoon Vanilla Extract (page 204)

....

For the mango soup

2 whole mangoes, peeled and cubed

1 cup chopped strawberries

Juice of 1 orange

Shredded coconut for garnish

....

For the ice cream

Combine all the ingredients in a blender and process on high until smooth, approximately 20 seconds.

Transfer the mixture to your ice-cream maker and process according to the manufacturer's instructions.

Once processed, place the ice cream in the freezer to solidify, approximately 10 minutes.

For the mango soup

Combine the mangoes, strawberries, and orange juice in a blender and process on high until creamy.

POPEYE'S KEFIR ICE CREAM

I make this ice cream at least once a week. I love it, and so does my family. Sadly, after reading this cookbook, my kids will know that there's spinach in the recipe, but your kids don't have to. Just tell them it's Popeye's ice cream. They'll think that's fun, and they won't taste the spinach.

Makes 12 servings

1¾ cup coconut milk or regular whole milk

1 cup frozen fruit (mixture of peaches, mango, and strawberry)

1 cup ice

¾ cup Kefir Cheese (page 17), preferably second-fermented

½ cup honey or Sucanat, or 3 to 4 teaspoons stevia

1 handful spinach leaves

Splash of Vanilla Extract (page 204)

Place all the ingredients in a food processor or blender and process on high until the ice is completely crushed and the ingredients combined.

Pour in an ice-cream maker and freeze according to the manufacturer's instructions.

PUMPKIN-KEFIR CHEESE ICE CREAM

I wrote most of the manuscript for this book on our boat. This particular recipe came to me one day when everybody at the lake was eating frozen custard while I was toiling away. To make myself feel better, I devised an ice-cream recipe with my favorite comfort foods, pumpkin and kefir. Pairing pumpkin and ice cream results in a rich, creamy concoction—and oh my word, it's so good! Deprivation can be a wonderful inspiration.

Makes 8 servings

2 cups heavy cream

1 cup fresh pumpkin purée or canned unsweetened pumpkin purée

¾ cup Kefir Cheese (page 17)

½ cup maple syrup

1 teaspoon Vanilla Extract (page 204)

½ teaspoon ground cinnamon

½ teaspoon ground ginger

¼ teaspoon Celtic Sea Salt

Pinch of freshly grated or ground nutmeg

1 tablespoon bourbon (optional)

Cinnamon-Toasted Pumpkin Seeds (page 182)

Place all the ingredients except the pumpkin seeds in a blender and process on high for 20 seconds. Pour the mixture into an ice-cream maker and process according to the manufacturer's instructions. Immediately before serving, top with the pumpkin seeds.

KEFIR FROSTY

When I first made this kefir frosty, my family remarked that it tasted like Wendy's. My version does taste just like it, but you can pronounce all the ingredients. You can use any ice-cream maker to freeze it, and the newer models will make the frosty in under 30 minutes. It's supercreamy and comes with the added bonus of kefir.

Makes 4 servings

2 cups heavy cream

1¾ cups coconut milk

½ cup Kefir Cheese (page 17)

½ cup Sucanat or honey, or 5 teaspoons stevia

2 heaping tablespoons Dutch-process cocoa powder

2 teaspoons Vanilla Extract (page 204)

Place all the ingredients in a blender and process on high for 1 minute, or until combined.

Transfer the mixture to your ice-cream maker and process according to the manufacturer's instructions.

After processing, pour in four tall glasses and enjoy.

GRAPE KOMBUCHA SLUSHY

This icy treat is great in the summertime! I love ice-cold kombucha when the weather is hot, but making this slushy is even better. You can use fermented or regular grapes—green or red. They're all refreshing and fun!

Makes 3 servings

2 cups Bubbly Fruit-Flavored Kombucha (page 173)

2 cups Fermented Cocktail Grapes (page 119) or regular grapes

. . . .

Pour the kombucha into an 8-inch square pan and add the grapes.

Put the mixture into the freezer.

Once the edges begin to freeze (approximately 20 minutes), scrape the icy bits to the center of the pan with a fork, and return the pan to the freezer. Do this again in another 20 minutes or so. Repeat the process until you have a pan of icy kombucha slush.

When you're ready to serve, scrape the slush into three tall glasses.

KOMBUCHA FLOATS

One of my favorite discoveries came when I combined kefir and kombucha. I've spoken before about my love of bubbles, and this float takes frothy bubbliness to a whole new dimension. I love it!

A note before you begin: The float delivers the most health benefits when you use kefir ice cream, but you can substitute regular ice cream, if you wish.

Makes 1 serving

2 cups kombucha, any flavor

1 scoop Kefir Ice Cream (page 156)

Pour half of the kombucha into a tall glass and add the scoop of kefir ice cream.

Pour the remaining kombucha over the ice cream to get a frothy mix, but be careful that it doesn't overflow. Serve immediately.

MACI'S CITRUS SYLLABUB

A syllabub is a creamy dessert served in glasses. This delicious treat was created by my daughter Maci one Christmas after she found an old cookbook from the 1800s. She took one of the recipes as her inspiration, and added kombucha. The combination was a hit!

A note before you begin: This drink can be made with plain kombucha, but you can also kick it up a notch and use Bubbly Fruit-Flavored Kombucha (page 173). That's how I always make it.

Makes 2 servings

¾ cup heavy whipping cream

Juice of ½ lemon

Juice of ½ orange

½ cup Basic Kombucha (page 28)

Pinch of Sucanat or stevia, or dash of honey

Place the whipping cream into a large mixing bowl and beat with a wire whisk or a hand mixer until soft peaks form. Set the bowl aside.

Mix together the lemon juice, orange juice, kombucha, and sweetener in a separate bowl.

Pour the juice mixture into the heavy cream, folding just enough to blend the juice and cream. The syllabub should be thick and frothy.

Cover the syllabub with plastic wrap and place in the refrigerator to chill before spooning into individual glasses for serving.

CHAPTER TWELVE

Beverages

One of the best things we can do to change the world is to consume healthy foods and drinks. As consumers, we vote for the foods and beverages we want with our hard-earned dollars. We can send a message to the market that we want healthier choices by spending our money wisely. Skip the chemical-loaded, nutrient-empty beverages on the supermarket shelves, and enjoy these wholesome and delicious homemade beverages instead.

COCONUT KEFIR SODA

Coconut kefir is loaded with probiotics, minerals, vitamins, antioxidants, amino acids, and enzymes. It's a wonderful alternative to store-bought sodas, and it tastes delicious. Plus, you can add all sorts of other refreshing flavors to this—a twist of lime, fresh ginger, or a squeeze of lemon.

A note before you begin: Make sure you use sturdy swing-top bottles (the caps clamp down) when making this recipe. You can repurpose beer bottles, such as those from Grolsch, or you can buy new heavy glass bottles that are specifically designed for brewing. Bottles bought at craft stores aren't as sturdy and may explode.

Makes 1 quart; 4 servings

4 cups young green coconut water

1 packet kefir powder starter culture

. . . .

Place the coconut water in a large bowl.

Add the kefir starter and stir until the starter has completely dissolved.

Transfer the mixture into 1-pint bottles, leaving 1 inch of headspace at the top of each bottle.

Clamp the caps closed, and let the bottles sit on the kitchen counter, out of direct sunlight, for 2 to 3 days, or until the soda is bubbly and fizzy.

Check the soda each day to see if it is bubbly enough for you. If not, let it ferment longer. A quick taste test will indicate when the soda is finished; it will be a little tart, not overly sweet.

Once the soda suits your taste, transfer the bottles to the refrigerator, reserving ½ cup of the soda mixture to make future batches, if desired.

A note on future batches: Using the reserved soda mixture, you can make up to 15 batches of soda before you have to open another packet of kefir powder culture. To make new batches, add **3½** cups coconut water to the reserved soda mixture, and ferment again. The fermentation process for repeat batches will be done in about one day. You will be able to tell when you need to use a new packet of kefir powder starter culture when the mixture will no longer carbonate.

Storage note: This soda can be stored in the sealed bottles in the fridge for up to three weeks. You should look at it every day and check the pressure by opening the bottle. Once open, the carbonation will start to decrease—just like store-bought soda.

STRAWBERRY-COCONUT KEFIR SODA

This beverage is so delicious that you'll want to drink it every day. It is fizzy and bubbly and full of flavor. It's a great way to get probiotics into your kids—it tastes so good they'll never guess it's also good for them!

A note before you begin: For a sophisticated touch, chill a glass or goblet in the freezer for a couple of hours before making the soda. When ready to serve, wet the rim of your glass and dip the glass in Celtic Sea Salt so only the outside of the glass is covered.

Makes 1 serving

5 whole hulled strawberries, frozen

2 cups Coconut Kefir Soda (page 166)

Put the strawberries and coconut kefir soda in a blender and mix on high until combined.

Pour the blended drink into a tall glass and serve immediately.

Storage note: This soda can be stored in sealed bottles in the fridge for up to three weeks. You should look at it every day and check the pressure by opening the bottle. Once open, the carbonation will start to decrease—just like store-bought soda.

GRAPE KEFIR SODA

I was writing my book and the deadline loomed. I was working frantically and drinking a bottle of this grape kefir soda when I realized something about myself: I work better under pressure. It causes me to focus in a more intense way, and I'm able to shut out the world. We can actually find our strengths when the pressure is on. Fermentation is the same. One minute you're a grape juice and the next you're grape kefir soda, completely transformed.

A note before you begin: Make sure you use sturdy swing-top bottles (the caps clamp down) when making this recipe. You can repurpose beer bottles, such as those from Grolsch, or you can buy new heavy glass bottles that are specifically designed for brewing. Bottles bought at craft stores aren't as sturdy and may explode.

Makes 1 quart; 4 servings

1 packet kefir culture starter powder

2 cups organic grape juice

....

Place the starter in 2 cups of filtered water and mix until the starter has dissolved.

Mix in the grape juice.

Transfer the mixture into 1-pint bottles, leaving 1 inch of headspace at the top of each bottle.

Clamp the caps closed and let the bottles sit on the kitchen counter, out of direct sunlight, for 2 to 3 days, or until the soda is bubbly and fizzy.

Check the soda each day to see if it is bubbly enough for you. If not, let it ferment longer. A quick taste test will indicate when the soda is finished: It will be a little tart, not overly sweet.

Once the soda suits your taste, transfer the bottles to the refrigerator, reserving ½ cup of the soda mixture to make future batches, if desired.

A note on future batches: Using the reserved soda mixture, you can make up to 15 batches of soda before you have to use another packet of kefir powder starter culture. To make new batches, add 1¾ cups filtered water and 1¾ cups grape juice to the reserved soda mixture, and ferment again. The fermentation process for repeat batches will be done in one day or less. You will be able to tell when you need to use a new packet of kefir powder starter culture when the mixture will no longer carbonate.

Storage note: This soda can be stored in the sealed bottles in the fridge for up to three weeks.

ORANGEADE KEFIR SODA

This is one of the few kefir soda recipes for which I like to use kefir whey, because it gives this soda a little more tang, and I really like the flavor. If you prefer, you can use a packet of kefir powder starter culture or water kefir crystals.

A note before you begin: Make sure you use sturdy swing-top bottles (the caps clamp down) when making this recipe. You can repurpose beer bottles, such as those from Grolsch, or you can buy new heavy glass bottles that are specifically designed for brewing. Bottles bought at craft stores aren't as sturdy and may explode.

Makes 1 pint; 2 servings

½ cup Kefir Whey (page 17)

⅓ cup orange juice

2 whole dates, pitted

Place all the ingredients in a 1-pint bottle, and then fill the bottle with filtered water, leaving 1 inch of headspace at the top.

Clamp the cap closed and let it sit on the kitchen counter, out of direct sunlight, for 5 days, or until the soda is bubbly and fizzy.

Check the soda each day to see if it is bubbly enough for you. If not, let it ferment longer. A quick taste test will indicate when the soda is finished: It will be a little tart, not overly sweet.

Once the soda suits your taste, transfer the bottle to the refrigerator. Before serving, remove dates, if desired.

Storage note: This soda can be stored in the sealed bottle in the fridge for up to three weeks. You should look at it every day and check the pressure by opening the bottle. Once open, the carbonation will start to decrease—just like store-bought soda.

STRAWBERRY KEFIR SODA

This is such a great soda. It has a ton a flavor, and you'll have leftover extract to make lots more soda. This is really great in the summertime when fresh fruit is in season.

A note before you begin: Make sure you use sturdy swing-top bottles (the caps clamp down) when making this recipe. You can repurpose beer bottles, such as those from Grolsch, or you can buy new heavy glass bottles that are specifically designed for brewing. Bottles bought at craft stores aren't as sturdy and may explode.

Makes 1 quart; 4 servings

1 packet kefir culture starter powder

⅔ cup Strawberry Extract (page 206)

....

Mix together the kefir starter and strawberry extract in a measuring cup with a spout.

Pour the mixture into a 1-quart bottle, and then fill the bottle with filtered water, leaving 1 inch of headspace at the top.

Clamp the caps closed and let the bottle sit on the kitchen counter, out of direct sunlight, for 3 days, or until the soda is bubbly and fizzy.

Check the soda each day to see if it is bubbly enough for you. If not, let it ferment longer. A quick taste test will indicate when the soda is finished: It will be a little tart, not overly sweet.

Once the soda suits your taste, transfer the bottle to the refrigerator, reserving ½ cup of the soda mixture to make future batches, if desired.

A note on future batches: Using the reserved soda mixture, you can make up to 15 batches of soda before you have to use another packet of kefir powder starter culture. To make new batches, add just under ⅔ cup strawberry extract to the reserved soda mixture, fill the bottle with filtered water as in step 2, and ferment again. The fermentation process for repeat batches will be done in 12 to 24 hours. You will be able to tell when you need to use a new packet of kefir powder starter culture when the mixture will no longer carbonate.

Storage note: This soda can be stored in the sealed bottle in the fridge for up to three weeks. You should look at it every day and check the pressure by opening the bottle. Once open, the carbonation will start to decrease—just like store-bought soda.

BLOODY MARY KEFIR SODA

This is a wonderful way to get lots of cultured veggies. After your Bloody Mary is made, garnish it with all kinds of fermented vegetables—dill pickles, celery, carrots, even olives—and then eat them as you enjoy your drink. I've even rimmed the glass with celery salt.

A note before you begin: Make sure you use sturdy swing-top bottles (the caps clamp down) when making this recipe. You can repurpose beer bottles, such as those from Grolsch, or you can buy new heavy glass bottles that are specifically designed for brewing. Bottles bought at craft stores aren't as sturdy and may explode.

Makes 1 pint

½ packet kefir culture starter powder

1¼ cups tomato juice

½ cup clam juice

1 teaspoon Worcestershire sauce

½ teaspoon celery salt

Splash of hot sauce (optional)

....

Place the starter in ¼ cup of filtered water and mix until the starter has dissolved.

Put the cultured water, tomato juice, clam juice, Worcestershire sauce, celery salt, and hot sauce, if using, into a 1-pint bottle, leaving 1 inch of headspace at the top.

Clamp the cap closed and let the bottle sit on the kitchen counter, out of direct sunlight, for 2 to 3 days, or until the soda is bubbly and fizzy.

Check the soda each day to see if it is bubbly enough for you. If not, let it ferment longer. A quick taste test will indicate when the soda is finished: It will be a little tart, not overly sweet.

Once the soda suits your taste, transfer the bottle to the refrigerator, reserving ¼ cup of the soda mixture to make future batches, if desired.

A note on future batches: Using the reserved soda mixture, you can make up to 15 batches of soda before you have to use another packet of kefir powder starter culture. To make new batches, add the tomato juice, clam juice, Worcestershire sauce, celery salt, and hot sauce, if using, to the reserved soda mixture, and ferment again. The fermentation process for repeat batches will be done in one day or less. You will be able to tell when you need to use a new packet of kefir powder

HOLIDAY KEFIR SODA

I gave some Holiday Kefir Soda to one of my good friends and workout buddies, Jayme. This started a trend where I work out, and now everybody is making kefir soda. They all ask each other if they've had their "kefir buzz." This excitement inspired me to dabble with some fun versions of this soda—I love the original recipe—but now I've also made the soda using cranberry, apple, and pomegranate juices. They're all delicious.

A note before you begin: Make sure you use sturdy swing-top bottles (the caps clamp down) when making this recipe. You can repurpose beer bottles, such as those from Grolsch, or you can buy new heavy glass bottles that are specifically designed for brewing. Bottles bought at craft stores aren't as sturdy and may explode.

Makes 1 quart; 4 servings

1 packet kefir culture starter powder

2 cups cranberry-peach juice

1 tea bag mulling spices or 1 teaspoon mulling spices sealed in a tea bag

....

Place the kefir starter in 2 cups of filtered water and mix until the starter has dissolved.

Pour the cultured water and juice into a 1-quart bottle, floating the tea bag on top and leaving 1 inch of headspace.

Clamp the cap closed and let the bottle sit on the kitchen counter, out of direct sunlight, for 2 to 3 days, or until the soda is bubbly and fizzy.

Check the soda each day to see if it is bubbly enough for you. If not, let it ferment longer. A quick taste test will indicate when the soda is finished: It will be a little tart, not overly sweet.

Once the soda suites your taste, remove the tea bag, being careful not to tear it open.

Transfer the bottle to the refrigerator, reserving ½ cup of the soda mixture to make future batches, if desired.

A note on future batches: Using the reserved soda mixture, you can make up to 15 batches of soda before you have to use another packet of kefir powder culture. To make new batches, add 1¾ cups filtered water and 1¾ cups juice to the reserved soda mixture, top with a tea bag of mulling spices, and ferment again. The fermentation process for repeat batches will be done in one day or less. You will be able to tell when you need to use a new packet of kefir powder starter culture when the mixture will no longer carbonate.

BUBBLY FRUIT-FLAVORED KOMBUCHA

A couple of years ago a friend was in a bad car accident. He was in the hospital on a gazillion pain-killers and medications and was completely miserable. I suggested that his wife bring him some kombucha. It made him feel so much better that when he finally got home, he started making kombucha himself. Now he makes the best fruit-flavored kombucha I've ever had. You can use any flavor of fruit juice and get great results.

A note before you begin: Make sure you use sturdy swing-top bottles (the caps clamp down) when making this recipe. You can repurpose beer bottles, such as those from Grolsch, or you can buy new heavy glass bottles that are specifically designed for brewing. Bottles bought at craft stores aren't as sturdy and may explode.

Makes 3½ quarts; 12 servings

One recipe Basic Kombucha (page 28)

1 to 2 cups fruit juice, any flavor

....

Place the brewed kombucha in six 1-pint bottles, leaving about 2 inches of headspace at the top of each bottle. If desired, strain the kombucha through a coffee filter to help prevent another kombucha culture from forming.

Add 1 to 2 ounces of fruit juice per 12 to 14 ounces of kombucha, leaving a little headspace at the top of each bottle.

Clamp the caps closed and date the bottles, so you know when the second ferment began.

Let the bottles sit in a dark place for 1 to 3 weeks.

Check the kombucha after each week to see if it is bubbly enough for you. If not, let it ferment longer.

Once the kombucha suits your taste, transfer the bottles to the refrigerator.

Storage note: This kombucha can be stored in the sealed bottles in the fridge for up to one year, but it will turn to vinegar over time. It is still fine to drink, but might be put to better use as vinegar because of the sour taste. Once open, the carbonation will start to decrease—just like regular store-bought soda.

KOMBUCHA ICED LECHE

This drink has a supercreamy, frothy head. It will also put everybody in a party mood! It's similar to an Italian soda, but it's more tart. I love it in the afternoon for a pick-me-up.

Makes 1 serving

1 cup Bubbly Fruit-Flavored Kombucha (page 173)

½ cup crushed ice

¼ cup coconut milk

1 teaspoon honey or Sucanat, or 1 to 2 packets stevia

....

Place all the ingredients in a blender and mix on high speed until very frothy, 30 seconds to 1 minute. Pour in a tall glass and serve immediately.

MARGARITA KOMBUCHA

I don't drink alcoholic beverages, but I've always loved the look of margaritas with their special glasses and salt-covered rims. And thanks to my daughter Maci, who came up with this recipe, I now have a great alternative to a tequila margarita that's delicious and healthy. And heck, with my pretty glass and a little sea salt on the rim, I'm not missing out on anything.

A note before you begin: Make sure you use sturdy swing-top bottles (the caps clamp down) when making this recipe. You can repurpose beer bottles, such as those from Grolsch, or you can buy new heavy glass bottles that are specifically designed for brewing. Bottles bought at craft stores aren't as sturdy and may explode.

Makes 1 pint; 2 servings

15 ounces Basic Kombucha (page 28)

2 tablespoons lime juice

1 tablespoon honey

1 teaspoon Celtic Sea Salt

Place all the ingredients in a bottle, leaving a little headspace at the top of the bottle.

Clamp the cap closed and date the bottle, so you know when the second ferment began.

Let the kombucha sit on your kitchen counter, out of direct sunlight, for 1 to 3 weeks.

Check the kombucha after each week to see if it is bubbly enough for you. If not, let it ferment longer.

Once the kombucha suits your taste, transfer the bottle to the refrigerator.

Storage note: This kombucha can be stored in the sealed bottle in the fridge for up to one year, but it will turn to vinegar over time. It is still fine to drink, but might be put to better use as vinegar because of the sour taste. Once open, the carbonation will start to decrease—just like store-bought soda.

COFFEE KOMBUCHA

One of my daughter Maci's favorite experiments has been making this coffee kombucha. It gives you the benefits of kombucha's probiotics plus the kick of coffee's caffeine. You can't ask for anything more. Second-generation fermenters come up with some of the best stuff.

A note before you begin: Make sure you use sturdy swing-top bottles (the caps clamp down) when making this recipe. You can repurpose beer bottles, such as those from Grolsch, or you can buy new heavy glass bottles that are specifically designed for brewing. Bottles bought at craft stores aren't as sturdy and may explode.

Makes 3 quarts; six 1-pint bottles

3 quarts (12 cups) freshly brewed organic coffee

1 cup sugar or Sucanat

1 cup Basic Kombucha (page 28)

1 SCOBY culture

....

As soon as the coffee has finished brewing, add the sugar and stir until it has dissolved. Set aside.

Once the coffee mixture has cooled, add the kombucha and SCOBY.

Place the mixture in a glass or ceramic container, and cover the jar with a cloth towel, secured with a tight rubber band.

Allow the jar to sit undisturbed at room temperature out of direct sunlight for 3 to 7 days.

Once the coffee kombucha suits your taste, pour the mixture into bottles, leaving a bit of headspace at the top of each bottle.

Clamp the caps closed and transfer the bottles to the refrigerator, reserving 1 cup of the coffee kombucha for making the next batch, if you like.

A note on future batches: When you make your second batch, you can use one cup of the coffee kombucha instead of the original kombucha. This will give it even more kick.

Storage note: This kombucha can be stored in the sealed bottles in the refrigerator for up to three months.

ICED KOFFUCA LATTE

This is creamy and bubbly, similar to an iced latte, but so much better for you. Iced lattes from the store are loaded with sugar and caffeine; this drink has a lot less, plus it gives you the added bonus of kefir.

A note before you begin: I like to make this drink using kefir because of all the health benefits, but you can also use milk, cream, or coconut milk if you wish.

Makes 1 serving

1 cup Coffee Kombucha (page 176)

1 cup ice

¼ cup Basic Kefir (page 15)

Honey, Sucanat, or stevia to taste

....

Place all the ingredients in a blender and mix on high until well blended.

Pour into a tall glass and enjoy.

ROOT BEER KOMBUCHA

The first part of this recipe makes a root beer extract that works perfectly for flavoring kombucha. You can also use this extract to make kefir soda. My favorite thing to do with root beer kombucha is to make a kombucha float with Kefir Ice Cream (page 156). To die for!!

A note before you begin: Make sure you use sturdy swing-top bottles (the caps clamp down) when making this recipe. You can repurpose beer bottles, such as those from Grolsch, or you can buy new heavy glass bottles that are specifically designed for brewing. Bottles bought at craft stores aren't as sturdy and may explode.

Makes 1 gallon; eight 1-pint bottles

For the root beer extract

1⅓ cups raisins

¾ cup boiling water

½ ounce dried sassafras bark*

3¾ cups Sucanat

....

For the flavored kombucha

14 cups Basic Kombucha (page 28)

....

For the root beer extract

Place the raisins in a bowl and pour the boiling water over them and let steep.

Pour 2 quarts of filtered water into a large saucepan over medium heat.

Place the sassafras bark into tea bags or closely woven cheesecloth and tie the bags with cooking string. Add it to the water.

As the water heats, stir in the Sucanat, adding about a ½ cup at a time. (Don't drop it all in at once!)

Simmer the mixture, uncovered, for 40 minutes.

Remove the saucepan from the heat; then remove the sassafras.

Strain the raisin water into the brew, and let it cool for at least 30 minutes.

For the flavored kombucha

After the root beer extract has cooled, pour about 14 ounces of kombucha into each 1-pint bottle.

Add about 2 ounces of the root beer extract to each bottle, adjusting the flavor to your liking and leaving a little headspace at the top of each bottle.

Clamp the caps closed, and date the bottles, so you know when the second ferment began.

Let the kombucha sit in a dark place for 1 to 3 weeks.

Check the kombucha after each week to see if it is bubbly enough for you. If not, let it ferment longer.

Once the kombucha suits your taste, transfer the bottles to the refrigerator.

Storage note: This kombucha can be stored in the sealed bottles in the fridge for up to one year, but it will turn to vinegar over time. It is still fine to drink, but might be put to better use as vinegar because of the sour taste. Once open, the carbonation will start to decrease—just like store-bought soda. The extra root beer extract can be stored in a sealed bottle in the fridge for up to two months.

* The root beer extract made in this recipe uses sassafras bark, which has been the subject of much controversy and many FDA warnings. Just so you know, these warnings were brought about by studies in which lab rats were fed huge amounts of sassafras, much more than you would normally ingest. In fact, when consumed in small amounts, sassafras has actually been shown to have protective qualities.

COCONUT KEFIR EGGNOG

I have an eggnog addiction. I wait all year for Christmastime, so I can justify drinking eggnog every day. And now that I've found a way to make kefir eggnog with stevia, thus eliminating the sugar, all my guilt has vanished.

A note before you begin: This recipe calls for consuming raw eggs, and people with compromised immune systems should not do so. For those of you who do choose to make the eggnog, I recommend using the freshest eggs possible. The best choice is to get your eggs directly from a farm or a reliable vendor at a farmers' market, but eggs from cage-free, pasture-raised chickens, which are sold in most grocery stores, are also generally safe.

Makes 6 cups

3½ cups coconut milk

1 cup Basic Kefir (page 15)

¼ cup Rum-Vanilla Extract (page 205) or ¼ cup rum

4 egg yolks

4 packets stevia

1 teaspoon almond extract

1 cup heavy whipping cream

Grated nutmeg for garnish

Place the coconut milk, kefir, rum vanilla, egg yolks, stevia, and almond extract in the blender and mix on high for 15 seconds.

Transfer the mixture into a bowl with a lid (or use plastic wrap).

Cover and chill the nog for at least 1 hour.

Whip the cream using a hand mixer on high speed until stiff peaks form when the beaters are lifted.

Fold the whipped cream into the chilled eggnog.

To serve, pour the eggnog into glasses and sprinkle with grated nutmeg.

Storage note: This eggnog can be stored in a sealed airtight container in the fridge for up to three weeks.

CHAPTER THIRTEEN

Condiments, Dressings, Flavorings, and Pickles

There is an easy way you can eat cultured foods every day—simply replace your standard condiments with cultured versions of them. There are recipes for almost every kind of condiment you can think of in this section. We use them so fast at my house that I make a lot of these on a regular basis. Make these recipes a part of your routine, and you'll discover how easy it is to adopt a cultured foods life. Kombucha Mayonnaise (page 186), Kefir Whipped Cream (page 183), and Kefir Ranch Dressing (page 189) are some of my must-haves, and they're in my refrigerator all the time, fermented jars of goodness disguised as condiments. I'd love to hear which of these recipes become your favorites.

CINNAMON-TOASTED PUMPKIN SEEDS

I use these pumpkin seeds on everything—soups, salads, sweet potatoes, and even ice cream. Oh, and bananas roasted on the grill with pumpkin seeds, honey, and cinnamon—to die for. But to be honest, most of the time these seeds don't make it into other dishes; they're just too good of a treat on their own. Even though they're not made with any cultured foods, they can be used with so many of the dishes in this book that I just had to include them.

Makes 1 cup; 6 servings

1 cup raw pumpkin seeds

2 teaspoons Sucanat

1 teaspoon Celtic Sea Salt

½ teaspoon ground cinnamon

1 tablespoon butter, melted

Preheat the oven to 275°F.

Wash the pumpkin seeds by rinsing them in a colander until the water runs clear, picking out any remaining pieces of pumpkin.

Drain well and spread the seeds out on a baking sheet; pat dry with a paper towel.

Mix together the Sucanat, salt, and cinnamon in a cup.

Drizzle the melted butter over the seeds and sprinkle them with the Sucanat mixture.

Gently toss the seeds until equally coated, and then spread the seeds evenly on the baking sheet.

Bake the seeds for approximately 30 minutes, or until lightly toasted, stirring every 10 minutes and checking for doneness each time.

Remove the seeds from the oven and let cool before storing in an airtight container to preserve freshness. They will keep for a few days at room temperature.

KEFIR WHIPPED CREAM

This is now the only way I make whipped cream. The kefir keeps the whipped cream stable, which means that it doesn't deflate and get all runny. It's whipped cream with staying power!

Makes 2 cups; 20 servings

1 cup heavy whipping cream

Honey, Sucanat, or stevia to taste

4 heaping tablespoons Kefir Cheese (page 17)

....

Pour the cream into the bowl of a stand mixer and beat on low speed until the cream thickens just enough not to spatter.

Increase the speed to medium-high and add the sweetener.

Continue to whip until the cream starts to hold soft peaks when the beaters are lifted. Gently fold in the kefir cheese with a rubber spatula or whisk.

Storage note: The whipped cream can be stored in a sealed airtight container in the fridge for up to one month.

KETCHUP

Store-bought ketchup has a lot of sugar in it, so I was looking for a way to reduce the amount of sugar in ketchup since so many people love it. My ketchup is supereasy to make and has a lot less sugar—plus, it's filled with probiotics!

Makes 4 cups; 64 servings

3 cups tomato paste, preferably organic

½ cup maple syrup

½ cup Asian fish sauce

¼ cup Kefir Whey (page 17) or ⅛ teaspoon Caldwell Starter Culture mixed with ¼ cup water

3 cloves garlic, peeled and mashed

1 tablespoon Celtic Sea Salt

½ teaspoon ground cumin

¼ teaspoon ground cinnamon

¼ teaspoon cayenne pepper

Put all the ingredients into a large bowl and stir together until combined.

Pour the mixture into two 1-pint or one 1-quart jar(s), leaving approximately 1 inch of headspace to let the ketchup ferment.

Seal the jar(s), and leave on the kitchen counter, out of direct sunlight, for 2 days; then transfer the ketchup to the refrigerator.

Storage note: This ketchup can be stored in the sealed jar(s) in the refrigerator for up to three months.

SPICY MUSTARD

When I was a little girl, my grandpa would make me a sandwich called a *bologna trobie*. He lived in Nova Scotia on an island, and it seemed that all the locals knew about this sandwich, but I had never heard of it. It was made with bread, thick slices of bologna, sliced onions, and seasoned with coarse mustard. He would spread the mustard on thick, and I loved it. That's what I'm always reminded of when I eat my mustard. Just a note: This starts out superspicy, but it mellows after a few days of fermenting.

Makes 1½ cups; 24 servings

1½ cups ground mustard

2 teaspoons Kefir Whey (page 17) or ⅛ teaspoon Caldwell Culture Starter

2 teaspoons Celtic Sea Salt

Juice of 1 lemon

¼ teaspoon paprika

1 garlic clove, mashed (optional)

2 tablespoons honey (optional)

....

Place all the ingredients in a medium bowl and mix until combined.

While mixing, slowly add ¾ cup of filtered water to create a creamy texture. Add more water if you like mustard that is a thinner consistency.

Spoon the mixture into two 1-pint jars and cap tightly, leaving 1 inch of headspace to let the mustard ferment.

Let the mustard sit on your kitchen counter, out of direct sunlight, for 3 days; then transfer the jars to the refrigerator.

Storage note: This mustard can be stored in the sealed jars in the refrigerator for up to three months.

KOMBUCHA MAYONNAISE

This is the only mayo I use. The taste is delicious, and there are no chemicals or preservatives; store-bought mayo can't compete. This mayo is so easy to make—it only takes about four minutes and uses just a few ingredients—that you can whip it up whenever you need it.

A note before you begin: This recipe calls for consuming raw eggs, and people with compromised immune systems should not do so. For those of you who do choose to make the mayo, I recommend using the freshest eggs possible. The best choice is to get eggs directly from a farm or a reliable vendor at a farmers' market, but eggs from cage-free, pasture-raised chickens, which are sold in most grocery stores, are also generally safe.

Makes 2 cups; 32 servings

¼ cup Basic Kombucha (page 28)

2 large egg yolks

½ teaspoon mustard powder

½ teaspoon onion powder

½ teaspoon garlic powder

½ teaspoon Celtic Sea Salt

1 cup extra-virgin olive oil

Place the kombucha, egg yolks, mustard powder, onion powder, garlic powder, and salt in the work bowl of a food processor, and pulse until mixed.

With the food processor running, slowly drizzle the olive oil through the feed tube.

Process for 4 to 5 minutes until the mixture thickens and is the creamy consistency of store-bought mayo.

Storage note: This mayonnaise can be stored in a sealed airtight container in the refrigerator for up to three months.

KEFIR-PISTACHIO PESTO

I eat pesto on everything. I have it on sprouted pasta, sandwiches, and fresh sliced tomatoes—I've even eaten it by the spoonful. I'm not sure if it's the fresh basil or my love of pistachios that makes this version so irresistible. Scoop out cherry tomatoes and stuff them with this pesto for an instant appetizer.

Makes 3 cups; 12 servings

1 to 2 garlic cloves

1 cup unsalted roasted pistachios, shelled

24 fresh basil leaves, torn into small pieces

¼ cup chopped fresh flat-leaf parsley

½ cup extra-virgin olive oil

½ cup Kefir Cheese (page 17)

¼ cup grated Parmesan cheese

2 tablespoons fresh lemon juice

½ teaspoon Celtic Sea Salt

....

Place the garlic in the work bowl of a food processor and pulse until finely minced.

Add the pistachios, basil, and parsley, and pulse several times until blended.

Add the olive oil, kefir cheese, Parmesan, lemon juice, and salt, and process until well combined.

Storage note: This pesto can be stored in either the fridge or the freezer. To store it in the fridge, keep the pesto in a sealed airtight container for up to one month. To use the pesto, remove it from the refrigerator at least 30 minutes before serving and allow it to come to room temperature. When stored in the freezer, the pesto will keep for up to three months in a sealed airtight container. When ready to use, place the frozen pesto in the fridge overnight to thaw, then remove it from the fridge at least 30 minutes before serving to allow it to come to room temperature.

KEFIR HOLLANDAISE SAUCE

This is a lovely, rich sauce that I like to serve over eggs. It's also delicious with vegetables.

Makes ½ cup; 3 servings

5 spinach leaves

1 basil leaf

3 tablespoons Kefir Cheese (page 17)

2 tablespoons grated Parmesan cheese

2 tablespoons freshly squeezed orange juice

1 egg yolk

1 tablespoon melted butter

Place the spinach, basil, kefir cheese, Parmesan, orange juice, and egg yolk in a blender, and pulse to mix thoroughly.

With the blender running on medium speed, slowly pour the melted butter into the mixture to emulsify, about 3 to 5 minutes.

Cover and place in a warm spot until ready to use.

Storage note: Store any unused portion of this sauce in a sealed airtight container in the refrigerator for up to three weeks.

KEFIR RANCH DRESSING

My husband loves ranch dressing, but I hate the commercial stuff. Most of it is full of MSG and artificial ingredients. So I spent a long time trying to create the perfect ranch dressing for him. He's finicky, so when he liked this, I knew I'd hit the jackpot.

A note before you begin: In the ingredients below, I've listed a range for the amount of kefir to use. The only thing that this changes is how thick your dressing will be. If you like a thick ranch, use less kefir. If you want a thin dressing, use more.

Makes 1¾ cups; 28 servings

½ cup Kombucha Mayonnaise (page 186)

½ cup Kefir Cheese (page 17)

¼ to ½ cup Basic Kefir (page 15)

⅛ cup chopped flat-leaf parsley

1 large garlic clove, minced

1 teaspoon white wine vinegar

1 teaspoon Worcestershire sauce

1 teaspoon Bragg Organic Sea Kelp Delight Seasoning

1 teaspoon onion salt or dehydrated minced onions

½ teaspoon paprika

½ teaspoon freshly ground black pepper

⅛ teaspoon cayenne pepper

Mix together all the ingredients in a food processor or blender on high until the mixture is smooth and creamy.

Transfer the dressing to a covered container and chill in the refrigerator for at least 1 hour to let the flavors meld.

Storage note: This dressing can be stored in a sealed airtight container in the refrigerator for up to one month.

KEFIR-BLUE CHEESE DRESSING

This is an easy and delicious way to get kefir into your daily diet. Pour the dressing over a wedge of lettuce and garnish with chopped tomatoes and extra blue-cheese crumbles. Or whip up a batch for the Buffalo wings at your Super Bowl party.

Makes 2 cups; 32 servings.

Juice of ½ lemon

½ cup Kombucha Mayonnaise (page 186)

½ cup Basic Kefir (page 17)

½ cup plain full-fat Greek yogurt

1½ teaspoons garlic powder

1½ teaspoons onion powder

3 ounces crumbled blue cheese

....

Combine the lemon juice, mayo, kefir, yogurt, garlic powder, and onion powder in a small bowl. Stir with a wire whisk until well mixed.

Fold in the crumbled blue cheese.

Storage note: This dressing can be stored in a sealed airtight container in the refrigerator for up to one month.

GODDESS OF FERMENTATION DRESSING

A friend gave me this nickname and the accompanying definition—Goddess of fermentation, *noun*: A lesser known but highly significant mythological creature recognized for her wise and natural healing of mere mortals' sepsis following their loss of health by following the prescriptive practices of minor deities. My kids had it printed onto a T-shirt for me.

Makes 1½ cups

½ cup Kombucha Mayonnaise (page 186)

¼ cup Bubbly Fruit-Flavored Kombucha (page 173)

¼ cup Basic Kefir (page 15)

3 teaspoons granulated garlic

2 teaspoons extra-virgin olive oil

2 teaspoons balsamic vinegar

Combine all the ingredients in a bowl, and whisk until smooth and creamy.

Storage note: This dressing can be stored in a sealed airtight container in the refrigerator for up to one month.

KOMBUCHA-RASPBERRY DRESSING

This is a great light dressing for summer salads, especially those that contain fruit.

Makes 1 cup; 8 servings

¼ cup Bubbly Fruit-Flavored Kombucha (raspberry, page 173)

2 tablespoons raspberry jam

2 teaspoons Dijon mustard

2 teaspoons minced shallots

¼ teaspoon Celtic Sea Salt

¼ teaspoon freshly ground black pepper

¾ cup extra-virgin olive oil

....

Combine the kombucha, jam, mustard, shallots, salt, and pepper in a bowl, and mix with a wire whisk.

While whisking, steadily drizzle in the olive oil to form an emulsion.

Storage note: This dressing can be stored in a sealed airtight container in the refrigerator for up to one month.

KEFIR CROUTONS

These croutons are really easy to make. They taste buttery, and they're great on salads. You can also use them to dip into your Kefir Cheese (page 17).

Makes 24 rounds; 8 servings

1 cup plus 2 tablespoons of Kefir Cheese (page 17)

⅔ cup Sprouted White-Wheat Flour (page 42)

3 tablespoons butter

1 egg white, lightly beaten

Celtic Sea Salt

....

Combine the kefir cheese, flour, and butter in the work bowl of a food processor, and process until the mixture is smooth.

Roll the mixture into logs as wide as quarter coins, or bigger, depending on how large you like your croutons.

Wrap the logs in wax paper and chill for at least 1 hour in the refrigerator.

Preheat the oven to 375°F.

Remove the wax paper, cut the logs into slices about ¼-inch thick, and place them on a baking sheet.

Brush the croutons with the egg white and sprinkle lightly with salt.

Bake for 15 to 20 minutes until lightly browned.

Remove the croutons from the oven and allow them to cool completely.

Storage note: These croutons can be stored in a sealed airtight container for up to three weeks.

HOMEMADE APPLE CIDER VINEGAR

All vinegars are made with what is called *the mother*. However, most commercial vinegars are pasteurized, killing the mother and all the good bacteria. But homemade vinegars still contain the mother, alive and well, which preserves them and makes them taste fantastic. It's well worth making your own.

Makes 6 cups

1½ cups Bragg Organic Apple Cider Vinegar containing the mother

4½ cups good-quality apple cider

....

Place the vinegar and the apple cider in a 1-gallon food-grade crock or jar.

Cover the mouth with a clean kitchen towel, securing the towel with a string or rubber band.

Store the crock at room temperature (68° to 70°F) for 1 to 2 months.

Check the vinegar once a month by sniffing and/or tasting it. It will gradually take on a distinct vinegar smell, and you will notice a slight film on the top.

When the mixture tastes and smells like vinegar, pour it into airtight bottles, and throw away the culture.

 A note on future batches: If you would like to keep the process going, instead of bottling all of the vinegar, simply bottle just a third of it, and replace the amount you've bottled with fresh apple cider and start the process again. The fermentation for this repeat batch will take less time, so check it often. Mine has fermented in as little as two weeks.

Storage note: This vinegar can be stored in a sealed airtight container in a cabinet indefinitely.

RED OR WHITE WINE VINEGAR

One of the most common ways to make this vinegar is to empty leftover glasses or bottles of wine into your vinegar pot. The good bacteria in "the mother" will kill any harmful bacteria and make a rich and robust vinegar that you'll love. Save that leftover wine, and your vinegar will be better than you can imagine.

A note before you begin: Finding a red- or white-wine vinegar containing the mother can be tough, but many health-food stores have them. Look for unpasteurized vinegar with sediment at the bottom of the bottle. The label will say *unpasteurized* or *with the mother*. The brand I often use is Eden.

Makes 6 cups

1½ cups red or white wine vinegar containing the mother

4½ cups red or white wine, any variety

....

Place the vinegar and the wine in a 1-gallon food-grade crock or jar.

Cover the mouth with a clean kitchen towel, securing the towel with a string or rubber band.

Store the crock at room temperature (68° to 70°F) for 1 to 2 months.

Check it by sniffing and/or tasting it once a month. It will gradually take on a distinct vinegar smell, and you will notice a slight film on the top.

When the mixture tastes and smells like vinegar, pour it into airtight bottles, and throw away the culture.

A note on future batches: If you would like to keep the process going, instead of bottling all of the vinegar, simply bottle just a third of it, and replace the amount you bottled with fresh wine and start the process again. The fermentation for this repeat batch will take less time, so check it often. Mine has fermented in as little as two weeks.

Storage note: This vinegar can be stored in a sealed airtight container in a cabinet indefinitely.

DONNA'S DILLS

Pickles are a comfort food for me. I eat these special pickles most often when I'm stressed, which I didn't notice until my web guy pointed it out. Now it's a running joke. I can't tell you how many times he has told or texted me, "Go eat some pickles!" He knows they will calm me down. Why do pickles make me feel better? That's a mystery to me, but I can't think of a better comfort food.

Makes 1 gallon

1 packet Caldwell's Starter Culture plus 2 teaspoons sugar or fruit juice or vegetable juice, or ½ cup Kefir Whey (page 17)

3 to 4 pounds small to medium cucumbers

4 garlic cloves

6 tablespoons Celtic Sea Salt

3 tablespoons whole dill seeds

2 tablespoons whole coriander seeds

1 teaspoon whole mixed peppercorns

1 teaspoon juniper berries

1 teaspoon fennel seeds

½ teaspoon red pepper flakes

If using the starter culture, place 1 cup of water in a glass measuring cup and add the sugar or juice. Then add the culture and stir until dissolved. Let the mixture sit while you prepare the cucumbers—anywhere between 5 and 15 minutes. If using kefir whey, add it when the recipe calls for culture.

Cut the cucumbers in half and place them, flat-side down, on a cutting board; then cut into spears.

Place the cucumber spears in four 1-quart jars.

Drop 1 garlic clove into each jar.

Place the salt, dill seeds, coriander seeds, peppercorns, juniper berries, fennel seeds, and red pepper flakes in a measuring cup with a spout for easy pouring. Add the culture and fill the jars with filtered water. Mix until well combined.

Pour the spice mixture into the jars, making sure that the spices are equally divided.

Fill the jars with filtered water, leaving 1½ inches of headspace to let the pickles bubble and expand as they ferment.

because the pickles rose above the water, do not worry. Remember, this isn't harmful. Just scoop out the moldy pickles and push the rest back under the water.

After 3 days, place the jars in the refrigerator so the fermentation slows. The pickles are ready to eat at this point, but they will taste best after being in the refrigerator for 3 to 4 weeks.

Storage note: These pickles can be kept in a covered airtight container in the refrigerator for up to nine months.

SWEET FERMENTED PICKLE RELISH

One time, I made this pickle relish, stuck it in the back of the fridge, and forgot about it. A year later I found it and opened it. It was bubbling and tasted really, really good. The added honey makes this recipe unique, and it ferments like a fine wine.

Makes 1 quart; 32 servings

3 cups chopped cucumbers

½ cup chopped onions

½ packet Caldwell's Starter Culture or ¼ cup Kefir Whey (page 17)

½ cup honey or maple syrup

½ red bell pepper, seeded and diced

1½ tablespoons Celtic Sea Salt

1 tablespoon whole celery seeds

1½ teaspoons yellow mustard seeds

1 teaspoon turmeric

....

Mix together the cucumbers and onions in a large bowl.

Transfer the mixture into a 1-quart glass or ceramic container that can be securely sealed.

Press the veggies down lightly with a spoon to pack them.

Combine the culture, honey, bell pepper, salt, celery seeds, mustard seeds, and turmeric, and then pour the mixture over the vegetables.

Add filtered water to cover, leaving 1 inch of headspace to let the vegetables bubble and expand as they ferment.

Seal the container and let it sit on your kitchen counter, out of direct sunlight, for 3 days.

Check the vegetables every day to make sure they are fully submerged in the water. If they have risen above the water, simply push them down so they are fully covered. If any mold formed because the veggies rose above the water, do not worry. Remember, this isn't harmful. Just scoop out the moldy vegetables and push the rest back under the water.

After 3 days, place the container in the refrigerator. This relish is ready to eat now, but it tastes best after being in the refrigerator for 3 to 4 weeks.

SPICY ZUCCHINI PICKLES

If you're like me and you have your own garden, chances are that come August you have an abundance of zucchini that you're looking for inventive ways to use. This is what I do with a good portion of my harvest, and once the cold weather arrives, I'm so happy to have them. They bring a little bit of summer to the winter table.

Makes 2 quarts; 12 servings

1 pound zucchini, sliced into spears

4 garlic cloves

2 tablespoons Celtic Sea Salt

1 tablespoon dill seeds

2 teaspoons red pepper flakes

1 teaspoon black peppercorns

1 teaspoon coriander seeds

1 teaspoon mustard seeds

¼ teaspoon of Caldwell Starter Culture or 2 tablespoons Kefir Whey (page 17)

Place the zucchini spears, garlic, salt, dill seeds, red pepper flakes, peppercorns, coriander seeds, and mustard seeds in two 1-quart glass or ceramic containers that can be securely sealed.

Add the culture, and cover the spears with filtered water, leaving 1 or 2 inches of headspace to let the pickles bubble and expand as they ferment.

Seal the containers and let them sit on your kitchen counter, out of direct sunlight, for 2 days.

Check the pickles every day to make sure they are fully submerged in the water. If they have risen above the water, simply push them down so they are fully covered. If any mold formed because the pickles rose above the water, do not worry. Remember, this isn't harmful. Just scoop out the moldy pickles and push the rest back under the water.

After 2 days, place the containers in the refrigerator. These pickles are ready to eat now, but they taste best after being in the refrigerator for 3 to 4 weeks.

Storage note: These pickles can be kept in a covered airtight container in the refrigerator for up to nine months.

CULTURED PURPLE ONIONS

These are great on sandwiches and salads—and especially good on pizza. These cultured onions get a little spicier as they ferment, which is something I've also noticed with jalapeños.

Makes 1 quart

¼ packet Caldwell's Starter Culture plus ½ teaspoon sugar or juice, or 2 tablespoons Kefir Whey (page 17)

3 medium red onions

2 tablespoons Sucanat

2 tablespoons coriander seeds

1 tablespoon mustard seeds

1 teaspoon Celtic Sea Salt

1 sprig thyme

....

If using the starter culture, place ¼ cup of water in a glass measuring cup and add the sugar or juice. Then add the culture and stir until dissolved. Let the mixture sit while you chop your vegetables—anywhere between 5 and 15 minutes. If using kefir whey, add it when the recipe calls for culture.

Peel and julienne the onions, and place them in a 1-quart glass or ceramic container that can be securely sealed.

Add the Sucanat, coriander and mustard seeds, salt, and thyme.

Add the culture and fill the container with filtered water, leaving 2 to 3 inches of headspace to let the onions bubble and expand as they ferment.

Seal the container and let it sit on your kitchen counter, out of direct sunlight, for 5 days.

Check the onions every day to make sure they are fully submerged in the water. If they have risen above the water, simply push them down so they are fully covered. If any mold formed because the veggies rose above the water, do not worry. Remember, this isn't harmful. Just scoop out the moldy onions and push the rest back under the water.

After 5 days, place the onions in the refrigerator.

Storage note: These onions can be stored in a covered airtight container in the refrigerator for up to nine months.

FERMENTED GARLIC

This recipe is one of my daughter Maci's creations. She made it for her brother, who loved it and begged her for more. Fermented garlic is super-bubbly and can be used in a ton of recipes. This is a great way to preserve garlic.

Makes 1 cup; 16 servings

¾ cup garlic cloves, peeled

½ teaspoon Celtic Sea Salt

¼ packet Caldwell's Starter Culture or 2 tablespoons Kefir Whey (page 17)

Place the garlic and salt in a 1-pint glass or ceramic container that can be securely sealed.

Fill the container with filtered water, leaving 1 inch of headspace to let the garlic bubble and expand as it ferments.

Add the culture and seal the container.

Let the container sit on your kitchen counter, out of direct sunlight, for 3 to 4 days.

After 3 to 4 days, place the garlic in the refrigerator.

Storage note: This garlic can be stored in a covered airtight container in the refrigerator for up to nine months.

FERMENTED JALAPEÑOS

This is another of Maci's creations. If you like jalapeños with an extra kick, try these. They seem to pick up heat as they ferment. Just a whiff when you open the jar can clear your sinuses.

Makes 1 quart; 32 servings

8 jalapeño peppers, tops removed and sliced lengthwise

5 to 6 sprigs cilantro

½ teaspoon Celtic Sea Salt

¼ packet of Caldwell's Starter Culture or 2 tablespoons Kefir Whey (page 17)

....

Place the jalapeños, cilantro, and salt in a 1-quart glass or ceramic container that can be securely sealed.

Fill the container with filtered water, leaving 1 inch of headspace to let the jalapeños bubble and expand as they ferment.

Add the culture and seal the container.

Let the container sit on your kitchen counter, out of direct sunlight, for 3 days.

After 3 days, place the jalapeños in the refrigerator.

Storage note: These jalapeños can be stored in a covered airtight container in the refrigerator for up to nine months.

APPLE, PEACH, AND PLUM CHUTNEY

I eat this chutney when I have a ploughman's lunch—sourdough bread, a hunk of Cheddar cheese, some dill pickles, and a little of this maple-fruit chutney. This is a cold meal that originated in the United Kingdom, but I do deviate slightly from tradition: I replace the bottle of beer with a delicious bottle of kombucha. It's one of my favorite meals.

Makes 2½ cups; 16 servings

1 apple, chopped into small pieces

1 peach, chopped into small pieces

1 plum, chopped into small pieces

⅓ cup raw cashews

¼ cup maple syrup

¼ cup apple juice

½ teaspoon Celtic Sea Salt

1 sprig rosemary

¼ packet Caldwell's Starter Culture or 2 tablespoons Kefir Whey (page 17)

Place the apple, peach, plum, cashews, maple syrup, apple juice, salt, and rosemary in a 1-quart glass or ceramic container that can be securely sealed.

Add the culture and fill the container with filtered water until it just covers the top of the fruit mixture, leaving at least 2 inches of headspace to let the fruit ferment. Don't add too much water.

Seal the container and let it sit on your counter, out of direct sunlight, for 3 days.

After 3 days, place the chutney in the refrigerator.

Storage note: This chutney can be stored in a covered airtight container in the refrigerator for up to nine months.

VANILLA EXTRACT

One of the easiest things I've ever made is my own vanilla extract. Take a few vanilla beans and plunk them in a cup of vodka. Let them steep awhile, and voilà—you have vanilla extract. I make large quantities, so I always have it on hand, because I use it in everything—from ice cream and baked goods to sauces.

A note before you begin: Once you finish making the extract, you'll have some deliciously marinated vanilla beans, which you can use for all sorts of recipes. My favorite way to use the leftover beans is to scrape out the seeds and use them in kefir ice cream. Or you can use the seeds to second-ferment your kefir.

Makes 2 cups

2 cups vodka

4 to 6 vanilla beans

....

Place the vodka and vanilla beans in a glass jar or bottle that can be securely sealed.

Seal the jar and set it in a cool, dark cabinet for 7 to 8 weeks. The mixture will get darker over time and the flavor will get more intense.

Storage note: This vanilla extract can be stored in a sealed airtight container in your cabinet indefinitely.

RUM-VANILLA EXTRACT

This is simply a different version of my original Vanilla Extract recipe (page 204). It has a slightly different flavor, so I find that it pairs better with some foods than plain vanilla extract. I use it in Kefir Ice Cream (page 156) and Chocolate Kefir Zucchini Cake (page 148).

A note before you begin: Just like in the Vanilla Extract recipe, you can use the leftover marinated beans.

Makes 2 cups

2 cups rum

4 to 6 vanilla beans

. . . .

Place rum and vanilla beans in a glass jar or bottle that can be securely sealed.

Seal the jar and set it in a cool dark cabinet for 7 to 8 weeks. This mixture will get darker over time and the flavor will get more intense.

Storage note: This vanilla extract can be stored in a sealed airtight container in your cabinet indefinitely.

STRAWBERRY EXTRACT

I like to make my own fruit extracts because the flavor is unbeatable. You can make this extract from any kind of fruit or combination of fruits. I love strawberry-and-rhubarb or peach-and-mango.

A note before you begin: You will have leftover fruit to use in recipes like Kefir Fruit Dip (page 75) and smoothies, so store the leftover fruit in a sealed container in the refrigerator or freezer until you're ready to use it.

Makes approximately 1 cup

1 pound strawberries, chopped or sliced

1¾ cups Sucanat

....

Place the strawberries in a bowl and add the Sucanat. Stir until the berries are well coated.

Cover the bowl with plastic wrap and let sit for 12 hours at room temperature (68° to 70°F), stirring occasionally to dissolve the sugar.

Strain the strawberries, reserving both the liquid extract and the berries.

Place the extract into a bottle, seal, and put it in the refrigerator.

Storage note: This extract can be stored in a sealed airtight container in the refrigerator for a month.

AFTERWORD

Finding Your Harbor of Healing

As you begin this journey, it is my heartfelt desire that you find the joy in cultured foods that I have. These foods have been an incredible gift to me. I am continually amazed by how they affect people—both physically and emotionally—and how easy and affordable they are to make. The stories I've heard and witnessed inspire me, and the list of ailments from which people have found relief continues to grow and diversify. These living cultured foods seem to help more illnesses, conditions, syndromes, and diseases than I could have ever imagined.

I have often said that there is more going on in cultured foods than I could ever explain. And as my experience grows, I believe this even more. The magic of cultured foods has changed my life. I hope you will learn to love these foods as much as I do. Thanks for reading, and I am confident you will find your own harbor of healing.

RESOURCES

Ingredients and Equipment

I've included links on my website so that you can click and purchase starters for kefir, kombucha, cultured vegetables, and sourdough. There are also many other wonderful conveniences and accessories for making fermented food, including air-lock jars, brew belts, and nonmetallic strainers. www.culturedfoodlife.com

In the United States, Heal Thyself is a community of people willing to share kefir grains. Visit the site to find out if there is a source near you. If not, there are options for mailing. www.heal-thyself.ning.com

The Kefir Grains International Sharing Community is a worldwide source of live kefir grains. www.torontoadvisors.com/suppliers

I've found Mountain Rose Herbs to be a reliable source for dried sassafras bark as well as for organic spices and teas. www.mountainroseherbs.com

Additional Information about Cultured Foods

Websites

Cultured Food Life, my own website and blog, where I and an enthusiastic community are waiting to welcome you to the cultured food life and to share our experiences, knowledge, and recipes. www.culturedfoodlife.com

Donna Gates and the Body Ecology website are a great resource for education and learning about cultured foods. www.bodyecology.com

Sandor Katz, the guru of fermentation, is brilliant. His was the first class I ever attended on fermentation. There is much to learn from this man and his books. www.wildfermentation.com

The Weston A. Price Foundation is a nonprofit organization that helps people find healthy and life-giving foods. www.westonaprice.org.

Books

Bentley, Nancy Lee. *Truly Cultured: Rejuvenating Taste, Health and Community With Naturally Fermented Foods*. Two Pie Radians, 2008.

Campbell-McBride, Natasha. *Gut and Psychology Syndrome: Natural Treatment for Dyspraxia, Autism, ADD, Dyslexia, ADHD, Depression, Schizophrenia*. Cambridge, United Kingdom: Medinform Publishing, 2010.

——. *Put Your Heart in Your Mouth*. Cambridge, United Kingdom: Medinform Publishing, 2007. Both books by Dr. Campbell-McBride were written by a physician who walks the walk and talks the talk.

Carroll, Ricki. *Home Cheese Making: Recipes for 75 Homemade Cheeses*. North Adams, MA: Storey Publishing, LLC, 2002. I use this book constantly. It is a wonderful resource for home cheese making.

Clements, Jillayne, and Michelle Stewart. *The Diet Rebel's Cookbook: Eating Clean and Green*. Springville, UT: Cedar Fort, Inc., 2010. This book has a lot of easy recipes using sprouted flour and nutrient-dense foods.

Enig, Mary G. *Know Your Fats: The Complete Primer for Understanding the Nutrition of Fats, Oils, and Cholesterol*. Silver Springs, MD: Bethesda Press, 2000.

Enig, Mary, and Sally Fallon. *Eat Fat, Lose Fat: The Healthy Alternative to Trans Fats*. (Reprint edition.) New York: Plume, 2006.

Fallon, Sally, and Mary Enig. *Nourishing Traditions: The Cookbook That Challenges Politically Correct Nutrition and the Diet Dictocrats*. Warsaw, IN: New Trends Publishing, Inc., 1999. One of the books that changed my life many years ago. If you only buy one book, buy this one.

Gates, Donna, and Linda Schatz. *The Body Ecology Diet: Recovering Your Health and Rebuilding Your Immunity*. (Revised edition.) New York: Hay House, 2011. This is the second book that I found that introduced me to cultured foods. It changed my life and started me on the road to recovery. I will always be grateful to Donna Gates for this life-changing book.

Gumpert, David E. *The Raw Milk Revolution: Behind America's Emerging Battle over Food Rights*. White River Junction, VT: Chelsea Green Publishing, 2009.

Hayes, Shannon. *The Grassfed Gourmet Cookbook: Healthy Cooking & Good Living with Pasture-Raised Foods*. West Fulton, NY: Left to Right Press, 2005.

Katz, Sandor Ellix. *Wild Fermentation: The Flavor, Nutrition, and Craft of Live-Culture Foods*. White River Junction, VT: Chelsea Green Publishing, 2003.

Luque, Ana. *The Yogurt Diet*. Los Angeles: Salud Life, LLC, 2008.

Pirtle, Kathryne. *Performance without Pain: A Step-by-Step Nutritional Program for Healing Pain, Inflammation and Chronic Ailments in Musicians, Athletes, Dancers . . . and Everyone Else*. Warsaw, IN: New Trends Publishing, Inc., 2006.

Planck, Nina. *Real Food for Mother and Baby*. New York: Bloomsbury USA, 2009.

Prentice, Jessica. *Full Moon Feast: Food and the Hunger for Connection*. White River Junction, VT: Chelsea Green Pub-

Quinn, Janie. *Essential Eating Sprouted Baking: With Whole Grain Flours That Digest as Vegetables.* Clarks Summit, PA: Azure Moon Publishing, 2008. This is the woman who opened my eyes to the benefits of making and using sprouted flour.

Rubin, Jordan S. *The Maker's Diet.* Lake Mary, FL: Siloam, A Strang Company, 2005. Healed from Crohn's disease, Rubin used cultured foods to heal his body.

Schmid, Ronald F. *Traditional Foods Are Your Best Medicine: Improving Health and Longevity with Native Nutrition.* Rochester, Vermont: Healing Arts Press, 1997.

———. *The Untold Story of Milk, Revised and Updated: The History, Politics and Science of Nature's Perfect Food: Raw Milk from Pasture-Fed Cows.* Warsaw, IN: New Trends Publishing, Inc., 2009. There are wonderful recipes for kefir and yogurt, and a discussion of the benefits of including them in your diet.

METRIC CONVERSION TABLES

STANDARD CUP	FINE POWDER (E.G., FLOUR)	GRAIN (E.G., RICE)	GRANULAR (E.G., SUGAR)	LIQUID SOLIDS (E.G., BUTTER)	LIQUID (E.G., MILK)
1	140 g	150 g	190 g	200 g	240 ml
¾	105 g	113 g	143 g	150 g	180 ml
⅔	93 g	100 g	125 g	133 g	160 ml
½	70 g	75 g	95 g	100 g	120 ml
⅓	47 g	50 g	63 g	67 g	80 ml
¼	35 g	38 g	48 g	50 g	60 ml
⅛	18 g	19 g	24 g	25 g	30 ml

USEFUL EQUIVALENTS FOR LIQUID INGREDIENTS BY VOLUME

¼ tsp				1 ml	
½ tsp				2 ml	
1 tsp				5 ml	
3 tsp	1 tbsp		½ fl oz	15 ml	
	2 tbsp	⅛ cup	1 fl oz	30 ml	
	4 tbsp	¼ cup	2 fl oz	60 ml	
	5⅓ tbsp	⅓ cup	3 fl oz	80 ml	
	8 tbsp	½ cup	4 fl oz	120 ml	
	10⅔ tbsp	⅔ cup	5 fl oz	160 ml	
	12 tbsp	¾ cup	6 fl oz	180 ml	
	16 tbsp	1 cup	8 fl oz	240 ml	
	1 pt	2 cups	16 fl oz	480 ml	
	1 qt	4 cups	32 fl oz	960 ml	
			33 fl oz	1000 ml	1 l

USEFUL EQUIVALENTS FOR DRY INGREDIENTS BY WEIGHT

To convert ounces to grams, multiply the number of ounces by 30.

1 oz	1/16 lb	30 g
4 oz	¼ lb	120 g
8 oz	½ lb	240 g
12 oz	¾ lb	360 g
16 oz	1 lb	480 g

USEFUL EQUIVALENTS FOR COOKING/OVEN TEMPERATURES

Process	Fahrenheit	Celsius	Gas Mark
Freeze Water	32° F	0° C	
Room Temperature	68° F	20° C	
Boil Water	212° F	100° C	
	325° F	160° C	3
	350° F	180° C	4
	375° F	190° C	5
Bake	400° F	200° C	6
	425° F	220° C	7
	450° F	230° C	8
Broil			Grill

USEFUL EQUIVALENTS FOR LENGTH

INDEX

ACKNOWLEDGMENTS

First and foremost I would like to thank my husband, Ron, who is the strength and love of my life. He has supported me and encouraged me, and believed in me like no other. The million hugs he gave me while writing this book fill the pages unseen. He is in every recipe, because he tasted them all. He read the pages first, and I have discovered that with him by my side I can do anything.

To my sister Danette, who believed in me from the time I was little, to the time she encouraged me to write a book. Thank you for your encouragement and for telling me to do it! Always being there for me through the good times and bad. Helping me with organizing the manuscript and for being my best friend when I needed someone the most. I will never be able to repay you for all you have done, but I sure plan on trying.

To my web manager, Chris Johnston, who is the rock that has helped me build my website and business. I realize that you are more than a website manager, but are a trusted friend and someone who was invested, believed, and supported me. It is not every day that you find a genius to create you a website and then watch as his talents extend even to helping with the book. You have made me better each step of the way. Words cannot express how grateful I am for you. You're a treasure to me.

To Patty Gift. Thank you for your kindness, guidance, and the genuine warmth you have shone on me, in person and through e-mail. You are someone who is a lighthouse to others and have helped me find my way. I hope you can feel my heart when I say, "Thank you, Patty!"

To my editor Laura, who has pulled the best from me while editing this book. Your questions and excitement about my book helped make it three times the book it was. Your skills and expertise helped me, and I will forever be changed by this experience of working

To the wonderful staff at Hay House, Quressa, Gail, Dani, I wouldn't be here without you and I am so grateful not just for your expertise but for discovering just what extraordinary and kind people you are. I am so proud to be affiliated with you. It means so much to me. Thank you!

For Maci, Malonda, Dane, Jeremiah, who helped me with pictures for my book. They're beautiful. Thank you for adding so much to my book.

Shelley Hanna, for my graphic pots. Those pots that you designed are everywhere in my business, and I am crazy about them. The thing I love the most about those pots is the friendship that was born from them.

ABOUT THE AUTHOR

Donna Schwenk is the Kansas City Chapter leader for the Weston Price Foundation, a worldwide organization comprised of people dedicated to restoring nutrient-dense food to the human diet through education, research, and activism. She is continually teaching classes in the Kansas City area, to show others what she has learned. She has been making and eating cultured foods since 2002. The dramatic change in her health and that of her family has given her a sense of well-being that has been incredible. After years of research, life experience, and teaching classes to help others, it is her pleasure to share it with you.

Hay House Titles of Related Interest

YOU CAN HEAL YOUR LIFE, the movie, starring Louise Hay & Friends
(available as an online streaming video)
Learn more at: **www.LouiseHayMovie.com**

THE SHIFT, the movie,
starring Dr. Wayne W. Dyer
(available as an online streaming video)
Learn more at: **www.DyerMovie.com**

*THE BODY ECOLOGY DIET: Recovering Your Health and Rebuilding
Your Immunity,* by Donna Gates with Linda Schatz

*CRAZY SEXY KITCHEN: 150 Plant-Empowered Recipes to Ignite
a Mouthwatering Revolution,* by Kris Carr with Chef Chad Sarno

*MEALS THAT HEAL INFLAMMATION: Embrace Healthy Living and Eliminate Pain,
One Meal at a Time,* by Julie Daniluk, R.H.N.

All of the above are available at your local bookstore,
or may be ordered by contacting Hay House (see next page).

✳

We hope you enjoyed this Hay House book. If you'd like to receive our online catalog featuring additional information on Hay House books and products, or if you'd like to find out more about the Hay Foundation, please contact:

Hay House, Inc., P.O. Box 5100, Carlsbad, CA 92018-5100
(760) 431-7695 or (800) 654-5126
(760) 431-6948 (fax) or (800) 650-5115 (fax)
www.hayhouse.com® • www.hayfoundation.org

❋

Published in Australia by: Hay House Australia Pty. Ltd.,
18/36 Ralph St., Alexandria NSW 2015
Phone: 612-9669-4299 • *Fax:* 612-9669-4144
www.hayhouse.com.au

Published in the United Kingdom by: Hay House UK, Ltd.,
The Sixth Floor, Watson House, 54 Baker Street, London W1U 7BU
Phone: +44 (0)20 3927 7290 • *Fax:* +44 (0)20 3927 7291
www.hayhouse.co.uk

Published in India by: Hay House Publishers India,
Muskaan Complex, Plot No. 3, B-2, Vasant Kunj, New Delhi 110 070
Phone: 91-11-4176-1620 • *Fax:* 91-11-4176-1630
www.hayhouse.co.in

❋

Access New Knowledge.
Anytime. Anywhere.

Learn and evolve at your own pace
with the world's leading experts.

Listen. Learn. Transform.

Embrace vibrant, lasting health with unlimited Hay House audios!

Unlock endless wisdom, fresh perspectives, and life-changing tools from world-renowned authors and teachers—helping you live your happiest, healthiest life. With the *Hay House Unlimited Audio* app, you can learn and grow in a way that fits your lifestyle . . . and your daily schedule.

With your membership, you can:

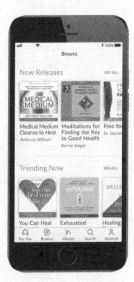

- Develop a healthier mind, body, and spirit through natural remedies, healthy foods, and powerful healing practices.

- Explore thousands of audiobooks, meditations, immersive learning programs, podcasts, and more.

- Access exclusive audios you won't find anywhere else.

- Experience completely unlimited listening. No credits. No limits. No kidding.

Try for FREE!